Emotions in Midwifery and Reproduction

To Tricia Anderson
1961–2007

Emotions in Midwifery and Reproduction

Edited by

Billie Hunter and Ruth Deery

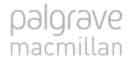

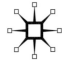
First published 2009 by
PALGRAVE MACMILLAN

Palgrave Macmillan in the UK is an imprint of Macmillan Publishers Limited,
registered in England, company number 785998, of Houndmills, Basingstoke,
Hampshire RG21 6XS.

Palgrave Macmillan in the US is a division of St Martin's Press LLC,
175 Fifth Avenue, New York, NY 10010.

Palgrave Macmillan is the global academic imprint of the above companies
and has companies and representatives throughout the world.

Palgrave® and Macmillan® are registered trademarks in the United States,
the United Kingdom, Europe and other countries.

ISBN-13: 978–0–230–54251–8
ISBN-10: 0–230–54251–4

This book is printed on paper suitable for recycling and made from fully
managed and sustained forest sources. Logging, pulping and manufacturing
processes are expected to conform to the environmental regulations of the
country of origin.

A catalogue record for this book is available from the British Library.

10   9   8   7   6   5   4   3   2   1
18 17 16 15 14 13 12 11 10 09

Printed in China

Contents

List of Tables and Figures

Tables

Figures

Foreword

Arlie Russell Hochschild

Opening the 17th International Midwives' Day on 5 May 2008, the convener told assembled celebrants: 'This year, around 136 million births will occur worldwide and the professional most likely to be present is a midwife. . . . In the midwife's hands,' she said, 'is the key to the future.' Citing findings from the highly reputed *Guide to Effective Care in Pregnancy and Childbirth*, Hannah Dahlen reported that 'when women with normal pregnancies were cared for by midwives, they were better supported, more satisfied with their care, had less medical acceleration of their labours, required fewer epidurals and episiotomies, had more normal births, and fewer babies that were underweight or needed resuscitation or admission to a neonatal intensive care unit.'[1]

How do midwives do it? They do it, the usual answer goes, by applying their medical knowledge, their technical know-how. And, of course, that's true. But a second reason for the midwives' extraordinary success, not mentioned at the international celebration, lies at the heart of this moving and important book. It is mastery of the complex art of relating to the entire personality and soul – not just the body – of a birthing mother. This calls on its own professional knowledge about how to succeed at emotional labour.

The essays in this book ask: what it is to become, not a friend, but '*like* a friend?' How does the midwife or other medical practitioner, extend a sense of real, full, compassionate *recognition* of a laboring mother or other involved persons? How, it asks, does the midwife help women face the disappointment of infertility, the fear of pain, the anguish of miscarriage, the extraordinary joy of giving birth? Feelings are 'natural' but our experience, recognition, and management of them is anything but. It is an art. The midwife supervises the passage of a fetus through a narrow canal into the light of day. But in a sense, through an encouraging tone of voice, a timely soothing hand upon an arm, a shared moment of silence, the midwife also guides an array of human feelings through a 'passage' as well. Parallel to the obvious intellectual and technical art of midwifery, this book argues, lays the equally important emotional art.

Troubling new trends are in motion, however, that make it harder for midwives to practise their emotional art. As this volume explains, neo-liberal policies driving privatization, deregulation and cut-backs in government funding have placed the focus on share-holder profit and Taylor-esque efficiency. Such policies have raised hours of work, reduced job security, lowered benefits, forgotten raises in pay, and routinised high turnover. They have moved the spotlight from *caring relationships* to the administration of abbreviated, fragmented, technical acts, estranging for mother and midwife alike. Drawing on the extraordinary collective experience of its authors, this welcome volume shifts the spotlight back to real care. Emotion work, its authors show, is real work, at time even *the* real work. This is the message of this book. Pass it on.

Sociology Department, University of California, Berkeley

Note

1 'Health Families: the Key to the Future', media release, International Midwives Day, 5 May 2008, http://wwwnswmidwives.com.au/events/internationalmidwivesday/tabid/99/Default.aspx, 7 May 2008. Hannah Dahlen, Head of the Midwives' Association of New South Wales, Australia, delivered these remarks.

Preface: Emotional Labour – What Do We Know and What Do We Need to Find Out?

Pam Smith

I was delighted to be invited to contribute a preface to a book on emotion work in midwifery and reproduction. Being a nurse with only some knowledge of midwifery, this was indeed an honour. I have, however, been a student of emotions in health care since my first days in nursing and this later evolved into the focus of my doctoral studies. During my early fieldwork I struggled to understand the nature of care, learning and the associated emotions, but I was fortunate to discover Arlie Russell Hochschild's work *The Managed Heart* early in my quest to investigate how student nurses learnt to care.

Hochschild's unique conceptualisation of emotion work and feeling rules has captured the sociological imagination and confirmed emotions as a legitimate field of study. A literature review[1] reveals that a wide range of disciplines and occupations have embraced the concepts, including bankers, social workers, call centre operators, doctors, nurses and midwives. There are also indications of a widening field in terms of emotional intelligence, emotions in organisations and leadership.

The notion of emotion management appears to resonate in whichever occupational setting it is considered, although the emotions to be managed vary and occupational feeling rules differ. Sources of emotional labour also differ considerably in different settings. Diverse studies have developed our understanding of emotion management, highlighting the particular nuances experienced by different occupational groups. For example, whilst some workers are expected to follow 'scripts' in relation to emotional display (such as the 'switch-on smile' of Hochschild's flight attendants), other workers experience much higher levels of autonomy (Bolton 2000).

Emotional labour is an under-reported, invisible component of service sector 'people' work largely undertaken by women. Emotional labour can also be used to explore the feeling rules within an organisation required to sustain relationships in situations that are often demanding and difficult. Hochschild describes emotional labour as 'The induction or suppression of feeling in order to sustain an outward appearance that produces in others a sense of being cared for in a convivial, safe place' (Hochschild 1983: 7).

For my research, *The Managed Heart* proved particularly important in giving a language to describe complex and nuanced situations, 'the little things' that would otherwise go unnoticed, such as making sure a patient's spectacles were clean.

But these 'little things' or 'gestures of caring' slip by unnoticed in the hustle and bustle of ward life (Smith 1992: 1). So why do we tend to describe them as 'little'? One explanation lies in the gender stereotyping of care as women's natural work which keeps it invisible and undervalued and on the margins of high-tech medically defined cure/care (Smith 1992: 2).

Ann Oakley, the feminist sociologist, admitted that, in 15 years of studying medical services, she had been blind to the contribution nurses made to health care, taking their presence for granted. It was only when she was a patient herself that she understood the significance of nurses and indeed attributed her survival to the intervention of one who emotionally lifted her spirits (Oakley 1984: 24).

As I began to analyse my data a new understanding leapt out at me. It was the language of emotional labour, the feeling rules, deep and surface acting, the work of face-to-face contact to produce feelings in others; and being supervised by ward sisters using particular emotional styles and setting the emotional tone.

During one such interview a student described the following incident:

> I've had times when I've been with another nurse and we've been changing the patient's bed and he's shouted at her or been rude or something. Well the procedure goes on as if nothing has happened. And when we've finished she just drifts off. And I actually go after her and say: 'Are you alright? I would have been very unhappy if he'd said that to me.' I think it is so important that we notice each other's distress so that we don't have to cry alone in a corner.   (Smith 1992: 8)

As this account demonstrates, nurses laboured emotionally not only for patients, but also for each other. The ward sister was the key person who set the tone for the caring climate on the ward. As one student explained: 'If sister cares then I don't have to take the whole caring attitude of the whole ward on my shoulders' (Smith 1992: 76).

In a keynote address to the Conference this book evolved from, Arlie Russell Hochschild expressed satisfaction that a wide range of scholars and practitioners had seized the opportunity to use emotional labour as a device to extend their conceptual and empirical thinking about emotions. Indeed, a review of the literature by Billie Hunter and Ruth Deery in the introduction to this book shows how emotional labour as an analytic device has proved vital for looking at the nature of caring.

It appears that emotion work is different for different occupational groups dependent on different clinical contexts and organisational set-ups. For example, in medicine, doctors' emotion management is influenced by the scientific approach to medicine on which their knowledge and skills are based. Medical students learn early in their training not to talk about their feelings either with each other or with their teachers, conforming to expected behaviours by learning to act 'as if' situations are neutral, resorting on occasion to 'gallows humour' (Smith III and Kleinman 1989). The resulting detachment helps them to distance themselves from death and dying, the fear of making mistakes and to handle uncertainty.

With regard to clinical contexts, Bolton (2000) shows how the emotional labour of the gynaecology ward goes beyond the associations of unrewarding work that is often seen as burdensome and emotionally costly to show how nurses viewed emotion work as part of the gift relationship (Titmuss 1970) which they freely gave to patients. In contrast to the medical students, the nurses described the use of humour in a therapeutic way for the benefit of patients by giving them the opportunity to have a laugh in the ward that was an 'emotionful place' and a 'woman's world'. They gave extra time to patients if they required it, expecting nothing in return, and then worked hard to enact professional feeling rules and present the image of a professional carer. A ward sister said: 'The essential basis of nursing is caring. You can't be a nurse if you don't care' (Bolton 2000: 583).

Within midwifery, also a 'woman's world', Billie Hunter found that it was managing the dissonance generated by the coexistence of conflicting ideologies of practice that was the key source of emotional labour (Hunter 2004, 2005). Research by Allcock and Standen (2001) and Hunter and Deery (2005) shows that students feel ill-prepared for the emotional demands of practice, and that little has changed since my study of pre-Project 2000 nursing students (Smith 1992). This insight is reinforced by Billie Hunter's personal contact with students at the Royal College of Midwives 16th Annual Conference for student midwives, many of whom told her they felt emotionally isolated and confused by conflicting feeling rules. Although nursing and midwifery curricula emphasise the importance of developing reflective practitioners, the role that awareness of emotion plays in this is far from clear (see also Deery 2005). The Standards for Proficiency for Pre-Registration Midwifery Education (NMC 2004) reflect a competency-based approach to the preparation of students that pays little heed to the emotional arena in which these students work. Similar tendencies are noted in nursing. Freshwater and Stickley (2005: 94) argue for the incorporation of emotions into the nursing curriculum which has been marginalised by the current emphasis on evidence-based practice, clinical outcomes and national standards. They conclude that making emotions explicit in the curriculum is an essential requirement to educate the emotionally intelligent practitioner. Whilst pockets of innovative educational practice for student midwives do exist (for example, the use of drama: see Chapter 12) these are few and far between.

In Chapter 3 Debora Bone draws on Hochschild's more recent theoretical developments in relation to the 'care deficit' that have led to the commercialisation of health and social care. Changes related to the 'care deficit' are seen within the emotional arena of the NHS where there has been a subtle shift from a public to commercial ethos embedded in financial incentives. This shift makes a study of the emotional labour of care particularly relevant, since Hochschild's original analysis was based in the commercial sector.

The changing nature of the health care sector therefore may bring new pressures, 'carrot and stick' incentives and mixed emotional responses as revealed by the results of the annual staff surveys undertaken by the Healthcare Commission (formerly the Commission for Health Improvement) (CHI 2003; HCC 2006). In these surveys, respondents described themselves as 'pilloried but proud', 'stressed but satisfied' at working in the NHS (Cornwell 2004).

A survey of NHS midwives reported they felt they had little or no say over their conditions of service, which interrupted their ability to maintain continuity of care and develop meaningful relationships with women and their families unless they gave extra time of their own accord which was not then valued by their managers (Ball et al. 2002).

Another aspect of commercialisation within the health care sector to consider is globalisation, which is manifest in an associated increase of migrant workers to the United Kingdom in general and nursing and midwifery in particular. Arlie Russell Hochschild and co-editor Barbara Ehrenreich (Ehrenreich and Hochschild 2003) refer to the global chains which bind women through complex family relationships to the economic imperatives of migration, as part of a 'care drain' which compensates for the 'care deficit' described by Debora Bone in Chapter 3.

The need to undertake new forms of emotional labour to manage the impact of migration on their professional and personal lives was evident in the findings of a recent study to explore the experiences of overseas nurses and midwives (Smith et al. 2006). The following quotations illustrate aspects of this experience:

> I was doing induction as a midwife all last year and I didn't finish. I was so frustrated as I really like midwifery with all of my heart but it felt like the midwives didn't want an outsider.   (an overseas midwife from South Africa)

> When I came here to work . . . one of my revelations in life was my emotions . . . if there are some problems in our house I don't need to bring them here to work. In my work there are bad days . . . and I don't need to bring them to the house.   (a Filipina nurse)

The ability of nurses, midwives and others to hold competing emotions while caring for patients and clients is at the heart of a number of studies which develop and critique the notion of emotional labour. McCreight (2005) considers nurses' use of emotions as a valid resource in the construction of professional knowledge while Mackintosh (2007) suggests they manage their emotions by 'adopting a working persona'. Theodosius (2006) proposes that emotional relationships connect individuals to each other, which in turn may assist them to contain their emotions (Hunter and Smith 2007).

To conclude, I have presented a variety of theoretical and empirical accounts of emotional labour to illustrate the complexities of emotion work and the importance of grappling with them at a macro and micro level. In recognition of these complexities, the Working with Emotions Network was established in 2000 to promote innovative research and practice in the field of emotions (http://portal.surrey.ac.uk/eihms_emnet). Through seminars and publications the network has created synergies between academics, professionals and practitioners.

The research agenda is set for more empirical testing and development of the concept, which will widen it out to psychoanalytic interpretation, politics and providing a platform from which the voices of users and carers can be heard.

Note

1   I would like to thank Dr Maria Lorentzon, Senior Visiting Fellow, University of Surrey for undertaking this review.

References

Allcock, N. and Standen, P. (2001) Student nurses' experiences of caring for patients in pain, *International Journal of Nursing Studies*, 3: 287–95.

Ball, L., Curtis, P. and Kirkham, M. (2002) Why do midwives leave?, http://www.rcm.org.uk (accessed 8 March 2007).

Bolton, S. C. (2000) Who cares? Offering emotions work as a 'gift' in the nursing labour process, *Journal of Advanced Nursing*, 32(3): 580–6.

Commission for Health Improvement (2003) 2003 national survey of NHS staff, Summary of key findings www.chi.gov.uk/eng/surveys/nss2003/index.shtml (accessed 9 March 2008).

Cornwell, J. (2004) Pilloried but proud, Jocelyn Cornwell on the NHS paradox: staff are stressed, abused and yet satisfied, *The Guardian*, 10 March.

Deery, R. (2005) An action research study exploring midwives' support needs and the effect of group clinical supervision, *Midwifery*, 21(2): 161–76.

Ehrenreich, B. and Hochschild, A. R. (2003) *Global Woman: Nannies, Maids and Sex Workers in the New Economy*. New York: Metropolitan Books.

Freshwater, D. and Stickley, T. (2005) The heart of the art: emotional intelligence in nurse education, *Nursing Inquiry*, 11: 91–8.

Graham, H. (1983) Caring: a labour of love. In J. Finch and D. Groves (eds), *A Labour of Love: Women, Work and Caring*. London: Routledge and Kegan Paul.

Healthcare Commission (2006) 2006 National survey of NHS staff, Summary of key finding, www.healthcarecommission.org.uk/healthcareproviders/nationalfindings/surveys (accessed 9 March 2008).

Hochschild, A. R. (1983) *The Managed Heart: Commercialisation of Human Feeling*. Berkeley: University of California Press.

Hunter, B. (2004) Conflicting ideologies as a source of emotion work in midwifery, *Midwifery*, 20: 261–72.

Hunter, B. (2005) Emotion work and boundary maintenance in hospital-based midwifery, *Midwifery*, 21: 253–66.

Hunter, B. and Deery, R. (2005) Building our knowledge about emotion work in midwifery: combining and comparing findings from two different research studies, *Evidence Based Midwifery*, 3(1): 10–15.

Hunter, B. and Smith, P. (2007) Emotional labour: Just another buzz word? *International Journal of Nursing Studies*, 44: 859–61.

Mackintosh, C. (2007) Protecting the self: A descriptive qualitative exploration of how registered nurses cope with working in surgical areas, *International Journal of Nursing Studies*, 44(6): 982–90.

McCreight, B. S. (2005) Perinatal grief and emotional labour: a study of nurses' experiences in gynae wards, *International Journal of Nursing Studies*, 42: 439–48.

NMC (Nursing and Midwifery Council) (2004) *Standards of Proficiency for Pre-registration Midwifery Education* (London: NMC).

Oakley, A. (1984) The importance of being a nurse, *Nursing Times*, 80(50): 24–7.

Smith III, A. C. and Kleinman, S. (1989) Managing emotions in medical school: students' contacts with the living and the dead, *Social Psychology Quarterley*, 52, 1. Special issue: *Sentiments, Affect and Emotion*: 56–69.

Smith, P. (1992) *The Emotional Labour of Nursing: How Nurses Care*. Basingstoke: Palgrave Macmillan.

Smith, P., Allan, H., Larsen, J., Henry, L. and Mackintosh, M. (2006) *Valuing and Recognising the Talents of a Diverse Healthcare Workforce*. June 2006. Report submitted. www.rcn.org.uk/publications/pdf/reoh_report.pdf.

Smith, P. and Mackintosh, M. (2007) Profession, market and class: nurse migration and the remaking of division and disadvantage, *Journal of Clinical Nursing*, 16(12): 2213–220.

Theodosius, C. (2006) Recovering emotion from emotion management. *Sociology*, 40(5): 893–910.

Titmuss, R. (1970) *The Gift Relationship*, London: George Allen and Unwin.

Acknowledgements

The initiative for this book evolved from the conference 'A Labour of Love?' Emotion Work in Reproductive Health held at the University of Huddersfield in September 2005. Ruth Deery, Billie Hunter and Mavis Kirkham, who were supported by Liz Senior in the Conference Office at Huddersfield, and student midwife stewards Laura Douglas, Selma Fitton and Linda Auckland, set up the conference. We are grateful to all those who attended and participated, especially Professor Sue Frost for opening and closing the conference, helping to make it such a creative, stimulating and friendly environment. We are especially grateful to Arlie Russell Hochschild, Mavis Kirkham and Debora Bone who encouraged us to build on some of the papers presented. We are also grateful to all the contributors who wrote their chapters in and amongst their other work and family commitments, especially those who had difficult personal circumstances. We would also like to take this opportunity to thank Sarah Lodge and Lynda Thompson at Palgrave Macmillan for their support during the writing of the book through to production, and to the anonymous reviewers for their encouraging and constructive comments. Inga Daniels provided secretarial support that was invaluable.

Billie Hunter and Ruth Deery

Notes on the Contributors

Helen Allan is Senior Research Fellow and Deputy Director of the Centre for Research in Nursing and Midwifery Education at the University of Surrey. She is also a nurse and registered nurse teacher and an invited speaker at European conferences. Helen is also a supervisor for a group of gynaecology nurses at the local NHS Trust and runs a monthly supervision group based on the Balint style approach. Much of her research focuses on infertility.

Kirsten Baker initially studied English and Drama and worked in theatre for several years before training as a midwife. She currently teaches at the University of the West of England, often using drama in the classroom. She is also the Director of Progress Theatre, a theatre company which comprises (mostly) midwives who devise and act. Their performances form the basis for explorations of midwifery practice and interagency working.

Susan Battersby is an independent midwifery researcher/lecturer and worked at the University of Sheffield as a midwifery lecturer until February 2006. She has a keen interest in infant feeding, particularly breastfeeding. She started the Sheffield Breastfeeding Initiative in 1989 and is still a member of the Sheffield Maternal and Infant Feeding Group. She also works as a volunteer breastfeeding peer counsellor at a children's centre in Sheffield.

Chris Bewley is Head of Department of Midwifery, Child Health and Primary Care, Middlesex University. She has been a midwife and midwife teacher since 1989. Her major area of research has been in the life experiences of midwives who do not have children, and those who have experienced loss of pregnancy, or other pregnancy-related loss.

Debora Bone is Director of the Cabrillo College Stroke and Acquired Disability Center, an adult-rehabilitation education programme. She was born and raised in the USA and studied nursing in Geneva, Switzerland. She worked as a maternity nurse in California for nearly twenty years before receiving her doctorate in Medical Sociology from the University of California, San Francisco, in 1997.

Ruth Deery is Reader in Midwifery at the University of Huddersfield. Her main work has been on the maternity services and women's health, with particular interests in service change and public policy. She is especially interested in women's experiences of childbirth and midwives' experiences of the organisation of maternity care. Her key interest at doctoral level was in midwives' support needs.

Fiona Dykes is Professor and Director of the Maternal and Infant Nutrition and Nurture Unit (MAINN) at University of Central Lancashire, in England. She focuses on socio-cultural and political influences upon maternal and infant health, and infant and young child feeding practices. She is domain editor for the international journal *Maternal & Child Nutrition*, and holds a range of other national and international editorial and advisory roles.

Nadine Pilley Edwards is an honorary researcher with Sheffield Hallam University and has been researching public participation through the experiences of women on Maternity Services Liaison Committees. She has been working with AIMS (the Association for Improvements in the Maternity Services) since 1980. Her book *Birthing Autonomy: Women's Experiences of Planning Home Births* was published in 2005.

Gina Finnerty is a lecturer and researcher based in the Centre for Research in Nursing and Midwifery Education at the University of Surrey. Her doctoral thesis explored the transfer of craft knowledge in midwifery practice and she continues to research with a focus on mentorship and coaching. Gina is a member of the Emotions Interest Group, led by Professor Pam Smith at the University of Surrey.

Billie Hunter is the first Midwifery Professor in Wales, based in the Institute for Health Research, Swansea University. She is also Visiting Senior Fellow at the University of Surrey, Chair of the Iolanthe Midwifery Trust and Chair of the All Wales Midwifery and Reproductive Health Research Forum. Billie's research uses qualitative approaches to explore how midwives work, and how this affects the care that women receive.

Mavis Kirkham is Emeritus Professor of Midwifery at Sheffield Hallam University. She has undertaken midwifery research and maintained a clinical practice, mainly homebirths, since 1972. Her research around birth uses several methods: historical, anthropological and surveys. Her research focuses upon women's experience of the work around birth and the childbearing years as mothers and as midwives.

Chris McCourt is Professor of Anthropology and Health at Thames Valley University, where she is based in the Centre for Research in Midwifery and Childbirth. She has worked widely on maternal health and maternity services and her research and teaching is mainly focused on culture and organisation of biomedicine, maternal and infant care, and social and cultural issues affecting women's health.

Ólöf Ásta Ólafsdóttir is Head of Midwifery Studies at the University of Iceland. She graduated as a midwife in 1978 from the Midwifery School of Iceland and in 2006 she was awarded a PhD from Thames Valley University in London with a dissertation entitled 'An Icelandic Midwifery Saga: Coming to Light – "With woman" and Connective Ways of Knowing'.

Hilary Piercy works as a Senior Lecturer within the Faculty of Health and Wellbeing at Sheffield Hallam University. She trained as a nurse and midwife. Her clinical, teaching and research interests and experience centre around the field of sexual and reproductive health. Her research has largely used qualitative methodologies to explore aspects of sexual health and service provision from the perspective of the individual.

Pam Smith is the General Nursing Council Endowed Chair in Nurse Education and Director of the Centre for Research in Nursing and Midwifery Education, University of Surrey. She combines sociology, health services research and qualitative methodologies to research the education and experience of healthcare professionals in the new NHS; emotions and care; leadership and organisations; student learning; patient safety; and the migrant health care workforce.

Trudy Stevens is Senior Lecturer in Midwifery at Anglia Ruskin University in Chelmsford. She trained as a midwife in 1975 and subsequently worked overseas in Nepal, Ascension Island, as well as in the Maldives where her experiences training traditional birth attendants taught her the meaning of midwifery. In 2003 she completed her PhD, which was entitled 'Midwife to Mid Wif: a Study of Caseload Midwifery'.

Introduction

Billie Hunter and Ruth Deery

Emotions were running high when, in autumn 2005, we sat in a hotel bar in northern England with a group of midwives, nurses, researchers and social scientists, to 'debrief' after the First International Conference on Midwifery, Reproduction and Emotion Work. Our discussions were excited and animated. The two-day conference had been a resounding success. For the first time, the emotional aspects of maternity care and reproductive health had been given an academic arena in which they could be explored and analysed. The conference had provided many opportunities for sharing and debating differing perspectives on the emotional aspects of midwifery, fertility work and gynaecological nursing. The discussions had been stimulating and challenging, generating new insights into the management of emotion in that most fundamental of experiences: the reproduction of human life.

And these insights had not been just of academic significance; it was also clear from the clinicians present that they had relevance for practice. A resounding 'take home message' from the conference had been that how we manage our emotions is important not only for the emotional well-being of health care practitioners, but is also a key component in the quality of the care which we provide. As we sat around the table, someone said, 'This is so important – we should put all these ideas down in a book.'

This book is the fruit of that idea. Many of the papers from the original conference are represented here, together with others that have come to our notice in the intervening period. Maternity care and reproductive health has also evolved in that period. UK maternity services have been the subject of growing professional and governmental concern, with workforce shortages (Ball et al. 2002) and low morale (Kirkham and Stapleton 2000; Deery 2003; Hunter 2002, 2004a) frequently cited as a major source of concern. Reproductive technologies are developing rapidly, bringing with them ethical dilemmas and complex decisions for all concerned. All these issues generate emotions: both for those at the receiving end of care, as well as those providing care.

How these emotions are *managed* is the subject of this book. Management of emotion is something that we do all of the time, in all aspects of our lives. For those who work with people it forms a significant aspect of our work. It is the invisible part of our job description, rarely appreciated when it is done well and authentically, but noticed when it is absent or insincere.

This book sets out to explore emotions in midwifery and reproductive health, focusing particularly on the challenges of emotion management for health care practitioners, especially midwives and nurses. It is the first book of its kind. This is surprising, given the obviously high emotional content in this area of health care work. As we will discuss later in this introduction, it is only within the past ten years that the significance of emotion in midwifery and reproductive health has been the subject of research attention. This book is certainly not meant to provide all the answers – indeed, many of the contributors in this volume generate questions rather than answers. There is much still to find out, and we hope that this book will stimulate debate and discussion, and lead to further research in this highly important area.

We will begin the introduction by explaining what is meant by management of emotion, including a discussion of the various terms used to describe this phenomenon. We will then provide an overview of emotion management theories, and consider how these have been applied to health care and in particular maternity care and reproduction. In the final section, we will provide an overview of each of the chapters, noting how they interrelate and drawing out the common themes identified by the various authors.

For readers who are new to the topic of emotion work we would advise you to read our introduction first and then 'dip' into the book according to your specific interest at the time.

What is emotional labour and emotion work?

The emotional aspects of work have only recently begun to receive detailed research consideration, due largely to the influential work of Arlie Russell Hochschild (1979, 1983). Since the *The Managed Heart* (Hochschild 1983) was published 25 years ago we have seen the rapid growth of research in this area. It is now acknowledged that work is as much an 'emotional arena' (Fineman 1993: 10) as any other part of life, and that in order to understand the complexities of work and organisations, we must pay careful attention to the 'feelings' aspect. However, it should be noted that emotion was not absent from previous studies of the workplace; rather it was relatively underdeveloped before the 1980s.

Early studies

Social scientists such as Goffman (1969), Hughes (1984) and Strauss et al. (1982) have all provided useful insights into the emotional life of occupations. Hughes (1984: 315), for example, considered that employees were not engaged in 'merely a bundle of tasks, but a social role, a part one plays in a drama' (p. 314). He noted that relationships between colleagues were of particular significance, observing that fellow workers 'can do most to make work sweet or sour' (p. 345). The emotional significance of relationships with colleagues is noted by many contributors in this book (see especially Chapters 4, 10, 12 and 13).

This conceptualisation of the workplace as a social drama has clear links with Goffman's work on the performance aspects of social encounters (used by Ruth Deery in Chapter 4, to assist her analysis of the 'performances' of community midwives). Goffman's (1969) analysis of social interaction in *The Presentation of Self in Everyday Life* focuses on the ways in which individuals attempt to control the impression they make, both as individuals and as team members in larger social enterprises. Although his work does not focus on emotion per se, expression or suppression of feeling is described as an integral aspect of impression management, as in the following:

> He can suppress his emotional response to his private problems, to his team-mates when they make mistakes, and to the audience when they induce untoward affection or hostility in him. And he can stop himself from laughing about matters which are defined as serious and stop himself taking seriously matters defined as humorous. In other words, he can suppress his spontaneous feelings in order to give the *appearance* of sticking to the *affective line*, the *expressive status quo*, established by his team's performance ... (Goffman 1969: 191, our emphasis)

This description implies that the individual manages their emotional responses in accordance with social norms regarding emotion, and that this is accomplished by a form of 'acting' by which 'actual affective response must be concealed and an appropriate affective response must be displayed' (Goffman 1969: 191). Appropriate emotional display is determined by social context. Goffman (p. 93) describes the different norms which operate in 'front region' areas (i.e. in view of the 'audi-ence') where 'politeness' and 'decorum' are expected, and compares these with 'backstage areas' where the illusion is suspended. This analy-sis of the emotion regulation required in order to ensure that emotional display is contextually appropriate has much in common with Hochschild's (1983) later, but similar, theory of emotion management (examples of which will be seen in Ruth Deery's chapter).

Finally, Anselm Strauss and colleagues (1982: 254) provided particu-lar insights into the emotional aspects of health care work, noting that there was 'more to medical work than its physiological core'. The phrase 'sentimental work' was coined to describe the emotional aspects of working on or with people. Different types of sentimental work were described and the invisibility of this work was noted, pre-empting the later comments of James (1989, 1992) relating to the lack of recognition of emotion work in nursing. It is notable that the concept of 'sentimen-tal work' is rarely given more than passing reference in the literature, in comparison with the enthusiastic response to the concept of emotional labour.

The work of Hochschild

It is the work of Hochschild (1979, 1983) that is credited with focusing specifically on the emotional aspects of work and, in particular, high-lighting the work that is undertaken in managing emotions. As will be seen, most of the contributors to this book draw on Hochschild's work within their chapters.

Hochschild's ideas have been adopted, developed and sometimes challenged by more recent authors (James 1989, 1992; Smith 1992; Fineman 1993, 2000; Bolton 2000). Her book *The Managed Heart: Commercialization of Human Feeling* (Hochschild 1983) was considered groundbreaking, as it drew attention not only to the significance of emotions in the workplace, but also to the work that is expended in managing these emotions.

This emotion management is conceptualised by Hochschild as 'emotional labour': 'I use the term emotional labor to mean the management of feeling to create a publicly observable facial and bodily display; emotional labour is sold for a wage and therefore has exchange value' (Hochschild 1983: 7). Emotional labour thus means the work that is carried out by individuals in order to control their own emotions, and those of others, so that they are appropriate for the situation. This is done in accordance with 'feeling rules' (Hochschild 1979: 563). These are the social norms relating to feeling and display, which determine not only which emotions should be *displayed* in a given situation, but also what should be *felt*. Hochschild argues that these rules generally go unnoticed until a mismatch occurs between what is felt, and what the individual perceives they should feel.

The identification of workplace feeling rules is well supported by evidence from other studies (Van Maanen and Kunda 1989; Smith 1992; Pogrebin and Poole 1995). These rules are particularly important in 'people work' as workers are required to interact with individuals who are experiencing extreme emotion of some kind. In these situations the level of emotional labour is raised: management expects workers to suppress their own feelings, however intense, in order to manage the feelings of others (Hochschild 1983). This has obvious implications for health care workers, who frequently encounter emotionally charged situations in their day-to-day work (James 1989, 1992; Smith 1992; Hunter 2002, 2004a; Deery 2003). The importance of emotional labour within health work is considered later in this chapter.

Hochschild makes a distinction between 'emotional labour' and 'emotion work': 'emotional labour' is performed in the public domain for a wage, and 'emotion work' takes place in the home, that is, the private domain. Emotional labour is subject to regulation by management. Hochschild contends that when workers sell their emotional labour to management, they become alienated because they are removed from their 'true' feelings. She proposes that emotions have thus become commercialised in order to meet economic imperatives. For example, in her empirical study of American flight attendants (Hochschild 1983), she observed how workers were trained to manage their emotions in order to comply with the corporate image of a friendly, personalised service. Flight attendants 'switched on' their smiles as they stepped into the public space of the aircraft cabin, saving their 'real' feelings for the backstage areas occupied by the crew. In this way, Hochschild argues, emotional labour becomes a form of capital, with workers 'selling their smiles' to employers.

In order to maintain the appropriate outer impression, workers make use of acting techniques. Hochschild proposes this can take the form of 'surface acting', where workers know that they are 'faking it', and 'deep acting', which she suggests entails working on altering inner feelings. From Hochschild's perspective, this latter form of acting is risky, as it may eventually lead to suppression of the true self. The worker ceases to realise that they are acting and becomes alienated from their feelings, with the danger of ultimate depersonalisation and burnout.

Recent thinking

More recent studies of public service work (James 1989, 1992; Smith 1992; Wharton 1993; Pogrebin and Poole 1995; Bolton 2000, 2001, 2005) have challenged some of these propositions. Rather than being passive victims in the face of management dictates, public service workers appear to have more autonomy in expression of emotion, and are thus not necessarily alienated from their emotions. These studies indicate that management of emotion is complex and likely to include both positive and negative emotions. It is also clearly affected by social and cultural context. Bolton (2000), for example, argues that when emotional labour is underpinned by a genuine sense of caring for another, as in nursing, it may be experienced as pleasurable work and there may not be negative consequences. Wharton's (1993, 1999) quantitative research identifies a number of factors that should be considered when assessing the emotional labour of an occupation: for example the level of occupational autonomy, the degree of job involvement and the potential for self-monitoring. She proposes that, when conditions are optimal, jobs that require emotional labour may bring rewards rather than burnout, and she challenges us to revise the negative frame in which emotion management is sometimes viewed.

A growing body of research has developed Hochschild's original concepts, indicating that the contours of emotional labour are even more complex than originally proposed (Steinberg and Figart 1999). Not only is emotional labour experienced differently in various types of work, but it is also experienced in diverse ways by individuals within an occupation. However, an inevitable outcome of this increased scholarly attention is the resulting lack of a consensus regarding the nature of emotional labour (Wharton 1999). Steinberg and Figart (1999: 13) provide a useful overview of current thinking. They identify several key characteristics of emotional labouring jobs:

- that they require contact with people, either within or external to the organisation;
- that the worker is required to manage their own emotions, but at the same time produce an emotional state in another;
- that, although the worker may control their own emotional reactions, there is also the potential for employers to control emotional labour through training and supervision.

There is also evidence of practical application of the concept: for example, the pay equity movement in North America has attempted to redesign traditional job evaluation frameworks to include emotional labour (Steinberg 1999). To do so, quantitative measures of emotional labour have been needed (Wharton 1993). Attempting to measure the components of emotional labour in this way is a radical attempt to increase its visibility and ensure adequate compensation for workers. The process is, however, necessarily reductionist and leads to the potential danger that emotional labour will become further commodified.

Management of emotions in the workplace is also linked to the notion of 'emotional intelligence' (Hunter 2004b; Goleman 2005). In his bestselling book, *Emotional Intelligence*, Goleman claims that emotionally intelligent people: recognise and manage their own emotions, motivate themselves, recognise the emotions of others and handle relationships in an effective manner. He suggests that individuals may have a high emotional intelligence quotient (EQ) in the way that they may have a high IQ, and that this EQ can be improved on in the way that IQ can be. His ideas have seized the public imagination, and can now be found in the language of human resource management, interpersonal skills and counselling training. Readers are encouraged to look at the original source (Goleman 2005) as well as critiques of this concept (see Fineman 2003) for further insights.

Clarification of terminologies

The rapid expansion of literature relating to emotions has resulted in differing usage of Hochschild's original terminology, which can prove confusing for readers. For example, the terms 'emotional labour' and 'emotion work' now tend to be used synonymously by many authors. Others make a case for using one term in preference to the other. In Billie Hunter's study of the emotional aspects of the work of midwives (2002, 2004a), she decided to use the term 'emotion work' in preference to 'emotional labour'. This was partly in acknowledgement that midwifery work is undertaken in both public domains (birth centres, hospitals) and also in the private domain of the home. It was also in response to her fieldwork, which suggested that midwives' work motivation differed significantly from that of workers in commercial organisations. For example, they often recounted working additional hours for no extra pay, and undertaking other types of unpaid work, suggesting that there are other factors at play in public service occupations than the relatively straightforward economic transactions described by Hochschild in her original analysis.

The differing use of these terminologies became evident when we read early drafts of chapters in this book. We made the decision that, rather than asking the contributors to conform to a standard terminology, we should recognise that different researchers may use these terms in varying ways. As you read the different chapters, therefore, you will become aware of these variations.

It is also the case that, particularly in health care literature, notions of emotional labour appear to have been merged with theories of caring. The concept has thus been redefined and broadened to include not only management of the practitioner's emotions, but also 'the nurse's use of self in attending to the psycho-social needs of patients' (Dingwall and Allen 2001: 65). That is, the concept has evolved to embrace all caring work that involves or generates emotion, rather than the effort needed to *manage* emotion. Whilst the work entailed in the therapeutic use of self is worthy of investigation and debate, it is clearly problematic to blur definitions in this way. This overarching concept of 'work that includes emotion' is also sometimes described as 'emotional work', thus adding another term to the pot. This semantic blurring has led McClure and Murphy (2007: 105) to comment that 'much of the emotional labour, emotion work/emotion management and emotional work literature are submerged in a semantic morass, which has led to further misunderstanding and misuse of emotional labour and emotion work in the nursing literature'. They recommend that a more robust concept be developed to accurately reflect the 'nature and complexity of professional nurses' waged and unwaged emotional work response behaviours' (p. 101).

Overview of chapters

This book is divided into four parts. Readers are encouraged to make use of the reflective questions at the end of each chapter, which are meant to facilitate further thought and encourage an increased understanding of research application to practice. The first part of the book, 'Emotion Work in Maternity Care', explores and provides important new insights into the concept of emotion work and its significance and use (or not) in maternity care settings. The perspectives of both providers and recipients of maternity care are considered. Chris McCourt and Trudy Stevens explore the significance of social relationships between midwives and women and provide a theoretical context to the meaning of 'continuity'. They draw conceptual links between two studies that examined different perspectives on caseload midwifery. Interestingly, the analysis and findings of each study mirrored the others. Knowing and being known, knowledge and confidence, in midwives and others, were found to be important aspects of social relationships. Reciprocal relationships were found to contribute to high levels of job satisfaction and reduced the potential for burnout.

Nadine Pilley Edwards focuses on the perspectives of birthing women, exploring the emotion work that they undertake in the context of what she describes as the 'industrialised, institutionalised maternity service in the UK'. She contends that birthing women are doing similar emotion work to that of midwives and that this is 'damaging rather than edifying to both groups'. She argues that whilst we persist in having 'dominant value systems that value measurable outcomes' in health care systems, emotion work will remain under-recognised and productivity and efficiency will dominate. Similarly, Debora Bone argues that market-driven health care and highly technologised obstetric care have led to a diminished quality of care for women in the United States. Epidural analgesia is used as an example of a post-modern solution to what she calls the 'contemporary care deficit'. She interviewed maternity nurses in northern California who provided antenatal and intrapartum care to women, asking them how they managed the emotion work involved in their work. These nurses described how 'techno-medical intervention' interfered with their care-giving processes, distancing 'mother and nurse from the deeper emotional connections' that may have been possible. The invisibility and lack of 'official' recognition of emotion work identified by Nadine Pilley Edwards and Debora Bone is discussed further by the next three authors in this section. Ruth Deery explores how a team of community midwives in the north of England managed and performed their emotions on a daily basis at work. The midwives had to calibrate their performances in order to meet organisational demands. Constantly having to change and calibrate their performances in this manner meant that little time was spent on their relationships with each other and women. Ruth Deery argues that if midwives are to retain their own sense of identity then emotion work in the UK National Health Service (NHS) has to be recognised and valued, rather than suppressed.

Fiona Dykes' study of midwifery work on postnatal wards in England provides new insights into the significance of time within maternity care, particularly focusing on how this affects relationships and emotion management. She highlights how a factory ethos and the mechanical clock have influenced hospital culture. This, she then argues, has a profound influence on the ability of someone to 'care'.

Fiona Dykes states that midwifery needs 'collective resistance and trans-formational change' in order to promote models of postnatal care where midwives and women can engage in meaningful relationships. Susan Battersby explores another aspect of postnatal care: the 'highly charged and emotional activity' of infant feeding. She challenges us to consider how emotional responses to breastfeeding on the part of the midwife may have an impact on the experiences of the woman. For example, she highlights how midwives may have ambivalent feelings towards supporting breastfeeding women, which stem from their own personal experiences of breastfeeding. Supporting women who choose to bottle feed may also create difficult emotional experiences for midwives, resulting in conflicting pulls of 'pro-breastfeeding rhetoric' and midwives' obligation to support women's choices.

The second part of the book, 'Emotion Work and Infertility' explores emotion work experiences in infertility settings. Helen Allan and Gina Finnerty highlight the gaps in emotional care of women who have undergone successful assisted conception. They also explore the litera-ture in relation to successful infertility treatment and question whether the emotional needs of women are best served through current practice of nurses, midwives and fertility nurses. Helen Allan and Gina Finnerty, like other authors in this book, highlight how organisational structures and professional identities may prevent integrated care. Chris Bewley replicated one of her previous research studies, with different inclusion and exclusion criteria, to interview midwives who were having prob-lems with aspects of their own reproduction. Needless to say, their expe-riences had profound effects on their own clinical practice. Given the considerable amount of emotion work that needs to be invested in midwifery, Chris Bewley provides several useful recommendations for the support of these midwives. Hilary Piercy's chapter is concerned with sexually transmitted infections, particularly genital chlamydial infec-tion, and how this can affect a woman's reproductive capabilities. She draws particular attention to women's anxieties about not being able to reproduce as a result of chlamydial infection. Hilary Piercy emphasises that the emotional burden imposed through fertility anxieties is likely to increase for women and health professionals, and needs urgent atten-tion from those responsible for service provision.

The third part of this book looks at 'Developing Emotional Awareness in Health Care Practitioners'. Billie Hunter explores the management of emotion in midwifery work as experienced by student midwives and those midwives in their first year of qualification in an area of South Wales. She draws attention to the midwifery ideal of being able to work in an 'affectively aware' (emotionally open) manner. However, as she found, this way of working was often unsustainable and midwives resorted to 'affective neutrality' (professional detachment) in order to cope with the demands imposed on them. She concludes that we need to enhance our understanding of how to manage emotions effectively in order to enhance the quality of care for women and their families. Ólöf Ásta Ólafsdóttir takes this discussion into a new arena, exploring how Icelandic midwives develop 'inner knowing' through their relationships with women. Using the birth stories of these midwives, she considers how midwives make use of connective ways of knowing (clinical skills and scientific knowledge) and an inner sensitivity to childbirth. She explores how inner knowing is linked to emotions, for example the emotional pressures created by this inner knowing in task-orientated and fragmented maternity care settings which do not value this form of knowledge. Kirsten Baker draws attention to the ways in which drama may be used to explore the emotional aspects of health care work. Using her experience as a midwife and as an actor for Progress Theatre she highlights how drama can facilitate 'safe and realistic exploration of the lived experience'. Her chapter presents some of the techniques and findings of this work.

In the final part of the book, 'Weaving It All Together', Mavis Kirkham pulls the threads together. She takes the reader on to a different level of thinking in relation to emotion work, drawing our attention to context and territory, autonomy, reciprocity, safety and trust, coping with the care deficit and learning emotional skills: key themes where change is needed because 'our emotional labour is an issue of quality of care for women and of occupational health for staff'.

References

Ball, L., Curtis, P. and Kirkham, M. (2002) *Why Do Midwives Leave?* Women's Informed Childbearing and Health Research Group, University of Sheffield.

Bolton, S. C. (2000) Who cares? Offering emotion work as a 'gift' in the nursing labour process, *Journal of Advanced Nursing*, 32(3): 580–6.

Bolton, S. C. (2001) Changing faces: nurses as emotional jugglers, *Sociology of Health and Illness*, 23(1): 85–100.

Bolton, S. C. (2005) *Emotion Management in the Workplace* (Basingstoke: Palgrave Macmillan).

Deery, R. (2003) Engaging with clinical supervision in a community midwifery setting: an action research study. Unpublished PhD thesis, University of Sheffield.

Dingwall, R. and Allen, D. (2001) The implications of healthcare reforms for the profession of nursing, *Nursing Inquiry*, 8(2): 64–74.

Fineman, S., ed. (1993) *Emotion in Organizations* (London: Sage).

Fineman, S., ed. (2000) *Emotion in Organizations*, 2nd edn (London: Sage).

Fineman, S., ed. (2003) *Understanding Emotion at Work* (London: Sage).

Goffman, E. (1969) *The Presentation of Self in Everyday Life* (London: Allen Lane, Penguin Press).

Goleman, D. (2005) *Emotional Intelligence* (London: Bantam Books).

Hochschild, A. R. (1979) Emotion work, feeling rules and social structure, *American Journal of Sociology*, 85(3): 551–75.

Hochschild, A. R. (1983) *The Managed Heart: Commercialization of Human Feeling* (Berkeley, CA: University of California Press).

Hughes, E. C. (1984) *The Sociological Eye: Selected Papers* (New Brunswick, NJ: Transaction Books).

Hunter, B. (2002) Emotion work in midwifery. Unpublished PhD thesis, University of Wales Swansea.

Hunter, B. (2004a) Conflicting ideologies as a source of emotion work in midwifery, *Midwifery*, 20: 261–72.

Hunter, B. (2004b) The importance of emotional intelligence in midwifery. Editorial, *British Journal of Midwifery*, October 2004, 12(10): 1–2.

James, N. (1989) Emotional labour: skill and work in the social regulation of feelings, *Sociological Review*, 37: 15–42.

James, N. (1992) Care = organisation + physical labour + emotional labour, *Sociology of Health and Illness*, 14(4): 489–509.

Kirkham, M. and Stapleton, H. (2000) Midwives' support needs as childbirth changes, *Journal of Advanced Nursing*, 32(2): 465–72.

McClure, R. and Murphy, C. (2007) Contesting the dominance of emotional labour in professional nursing, *Journal of Health Organization and Management*, 21(2): 101–20.

Pogrebin, M. R. and Poole, E. D. (1995) Emotion management: A study of police response to tragic events, *Social Perspectives on Emotion*, 3: 149–68.

Smith, P. (1992) *The Emotional Labour of Nursing* (Basingstoke: Palgrave Macmillan).

Steinberg, R. J. (1999) Emotional labor in job evaluation: redesigning compensation practices. In R. J. Steinberg and D. M. Figart (eds), *Emotional Labor in the Service Economy*. The Annals of the American Academy of Political and Social Science, pp. 143–57.

Steinberg, R. J. and Figart, D. M. (1999) Emotional labor since *The Managed Heart*. In R. J. Steinberg and D. M.Figart (eds), *Emotional Labor in the Service Economy*. The Annals of the American Academy of Political and Social Science, pp. 8–25.

Strauss, A., Fagerhaugh, S., Suczek, B. and Wiener, C. (1982) Sentimental work in the technologized hospital, *Sociology of Health and Illness*, 4(3): 254–78.

Van Maanen, J. and Kunda, G. (1989) 'Real feelings': Emotional expression and organizational culture, *Research in Organizational Behavior*, 11: 43–103.

Wharton, A. S. (1993) The affective consequences of service work: Managing emotions on the job, *Work and Occupations*, 20(2): 205–32.

Wharton, A. S. (1999) The psycho-social consequences of emotional labor. In R. J. Steinberg and D. N. Figart (eds), *Emotional Labor in the Service Economy*, Annals of the American Academy of Political and Social Science, pp. 158–75.

PART I

Emotion Work in Maternity Care

1

Relationship and Reciprocity in Caseload Midwifery

Chris McCourt and Trudy Stevens

Introduction

This chapter explores ways in which the organisation of midwifery care may be seen to affect the emotional work that is central to childbirth. It is drawn from a study of caseload practice that was implemented in the UK, following the publication of the Changing Childbirth report (Department of Health 1993), designed to support woman-centred care.

The traditional, Old English, meaning of the word 'midwife' is said to be 'with woman'. Such meaning and values are clearly held by midwives and the importance of being 'with woman' is strongly articulated by midwifery students and practitioners as a defining characteristic of midwifery. However, a number of studies have suggested a considerable gap between such core values and those revealed in much of midwifery practice. For example, ethnographic (Kirkham 1989) and observation-based (Methven 1989) studies have indicated that midwives in practice spend relatively little of their time in work that could fairly be described as directly supporting or working with women.

A key focus of our evaluation was whether the new model of care would actually be woman-centred in practice, and whether it was experienced positively by those who were *providing* care as well as those receiving it. A structured review (Green et al. 1998) concluded that while there was evidence of women's satisfaction with new models of care, there was little evidence on midwives' experiences; they questioned whether the importance of continuity of carer to women justified the possible 'costs' to midwives. A large-scale analysis of midwives' stress and burnout, however, found that high levels of both were associated with team rather than caseload midwifery (Sandall 1997).

In a study of emotional labour, Hunter (2004) found that midwives viewed the basic work of midwifery as a positive form of such labour, but experienced considerable distress through other, less anticipated, forms. These centred on managing institutional and work-related demands, intra- and inter-professional tensions and conflicts, and hier-archical and horizontal forms of oppression (see also Deery 2005). Such studies echoed the themes of a considerable wider literature on the nature of institutional work, on the experiences and behaviour of oppressed groups and on work-related stress and burnout. The study we draw on here offers a different perspective, indicating that midwives carrying personal caseloads experienced considerable job satisfaction and reward (Stevens and McCourt 2001, 2002a, 2002b, 2002c; Stevens 2003).

During our analyses it was noted that conceptual links could be drawn between the two aspects of the evaluation that examined the experiences of women and those of midwives. The first study explored women's responses to maternity care through a longitudinal survey and interviews; the second was an ethnographic study of the impact of the change on midwives. This chapter sets the analysis of each alongside the other and highlights ways in which each group's narratives echoed those of the other, particularly in relation to the emotional aspect of preparing for, and caring for, birth.

The key themes

The key themes identified in each analysis were set alongside each other, as shown in Table 1.1. We discuss these in turn, considering both the women's and the midwives' perspectives on each.

Knowing and being known

Knowing each other emerged as an important theme in both analyses and clearly held significance for the well-being of mothers and midwives. The women's accounts indicated that 'knowing the midwife' was more complex than simply having met the person more than once; it was about the midwife knowing them. This was not the same as the intimacy of friendship or kinship, since the relationship was circumscribed by the

Table 1.1   Women's and midwives' perspectives

Key theme	Women's perspectives	Midwives' perspectives
Knowing and being known	Knowing the midwife; *'my'* midwife; being known by the midwife.	Relationship with the woman; *'my'* woman; reciprocity.
Person-centred care	Care focused on me as a person; someone there for you.	Being a person not a role; personal orientation; being there.
Social support	Social support.	Support from partnerships and groups.
Reassurance, confidence and development	Reassurance, sense of confidence.	Confidence and development.
Informed choice, control and autonomy	Informed choice and decision making; sense of control (locus of control).	Autonomy; decision making; control over own work.
Holistic and flexible care	Flexible care, not a production line; time to listen and give care; place – hospital to community; medical and social care.	Time orientation; flexibility; place – with the woman; using all skills; integrated.

experience of maternity; midwives were not seen as friends but were often seen as *like* friends or *like* kin:

> . . . my midwife and myself got on well. She was like my family there. (Caseload care 116)

When compared with conventional care, the difference in relationship was illustrated by the pronouns used by both women and midwives: *'my'* rather than *'the'* midwife, and *'my'* women.

Such terms could signify some kind of professional territorialism or desire for control and, in attempting to be all things to all women in their care, might create a disempowering sense of dependency. However, their use here appeared to signify a sense of obligation and responsibility primarily to the care of the women on their caseload:

I'm definitely more in tune with the women that I look after and I certainly respect [the] women – because I know them and I'll do the best to help them make the choices they want – you know, to help them achieve what they've said to me that they're hoping from the birth.   (Caseload midwife 6)

The importance of being known was emphasised by some women for its contrast with a fragmented system where you could not be known, where who you were was forgotten, where your history had to be told over and over, where you did not feel listened to, except in a superficial way. One woman, for example, described wanting to tell midwives about the effect of domestic violence. She had hoped that someone would ask her how things were at home:

. . . and I would probably have broke down and let the whole thing out. But they've got a hard job to do as well so I must appreciate that, because there are a lot of women having babies.   (Conventional care 370)

However, she found that apart from visits to her GP, she saw different people every time, and was made to feel a nuisance if she tried to talk about how she felt. Nevertheless, the depth of relationship that appeared necessary before some mothers disclosed such intimate situations surprised the caseload midwives:

I was really shocked the other day when a woman reached 34/40 pregnant before she was able to tell me that she had been sexually abused. It would never have come out in the conventional service. As it was I could be sensitive to every nuance.   (Focus group of caseload midwives)

The emphasis on the relationship was equally important for the midwives, who felt they gained from the relationship with women in their care, rather than just giving. We suggest that this sense of reciprocity offered an important defence mechanism that helped prevent the 'burnout' that could be thought to be a danger of working in this way (Stevens 2003).

The midwives felt known – and valued; they talked about 'actually being a person again, not just a cog in a wheel', and highlighted the way women related to them as individuals. The implication was that they had not been considered and valued as people when working in the hospital service, merely pairs of hands to get the work done. They also considered that they used many of their personal skills in their daily work that they had not found utilised in the hospital system. No longer tied by the routines and immediate workload pressures that dominated hospital practice, caseload midwives reported being creative in their practice, responding to the needs of their women in a more imaginative way than they had experienced working in the 'confines' of the hospital. They were able to practise the 'art' as well as the 'science' of midwifery in a manner that drew on their individual skills and strengths, not just their technical abilities. This feature was facilitated by their sense of 'ownership' of their caseload in accepting responsibility for care provided.

Also, importantly, they felt that knowing the woman meant they were not constantly starting over, and they could understand more. Prior knowledge meant some things were easier – such as supporting the woman in labour:

> It's very easy to look after women in labour when you know them . . . Because you've got to build up this relationship with them, got to know them [and they've] got to like you. You've gone through all that by the time they go into labour. It's far easier . . . They are far more relaxed. (Caseload midwife 62)

Other issues could be more difficult, such as establishing limits to the care they should offer to a 'needy' woman. Nevertheless, this problem was recognised early by the midwives, who then learnt to define their role clearly in the early stages of the relationship, and to 'educate' their women, as they termed it. They also built up local knowledge and contacts, so that they could refer and connect women to other sources of social support. In many cases, the sense of relationship engendered a sense of mutual trust and obligation that was important to both the woman and the midwife:

> And they really do tell you things. Very deep things. Very personal things. But it does make it easier to look after them because you can actually see why they're behaving that way or going through it. (Caseload midwife 23)

The midwives also gained a sense of professional and personal satisfaction from feeling that they had seen a particular relationship through – the accepted conclusion being the end of postnatal care and the settling of the woman into new parenthood. Occasionally this proved longer-term as individual relationships were renewed in subsequent pregnancies, something warmly welcomed even when a childbearing experience had proved difficult. Recounting her experience of caring for a mother after a previous stillbirth, one midwife noted:

> She had two others since then and she's as happy as anything – because I went through that traumatic time with her and it helped her to grieve and it helped her to accept the other two pregnancies much more easily. Because I knew [what she had gone through] we could talk about it much more easily.   (Caseload midwife 21)

Such relationships may hold psychological benefits for both the woman experiencing such traumas and the midwife supporting her.

Person-centred care

For both women and midwives, the organisation of care appeared more person-centred. This was reflected in the orientation of the midwives' work and sense of responsibility, which appeared to shift from accountability to the institution towards accountability to the client and to the profession of midwifery. Autonomy of practice and expectation of continuity gave them space and time to get to know the particular circumstances of each mother; by recognising the individuality of each case the women became special because they were different and they demanded different responses. Emotions were engaged, but were 'worked through' by midwife and mother, not denied behind a professional 'mask'.

Person-centred care was highlighted by the importance attached to the phrases 'having someone there for me' and 'being there':

> . . . knowing that I could like pick the phone up and talk to someone on a one-to-one basis sort of, like really relaxed me and gave me the confidence to carry on.   (Caseload care 717)

In practice, knowing that the midwife was 'there for you' did not engender greater dependency; the women reported that they rarely called as they had the confidence of knowing they could, if they really needed to.

For the midwives the 'being there' was an idea that was closely linked to the expectation of continuity and the autonomy the midwives experienced. Their work with an individual held a greater significance because they knew they would be following through a case and had the power to influence the situation.

> During the booking visit you are investing time for the future. (Caseload midwife 8)

Providing continuity and having responsibility were seen to be cate-gorical in the midwives being able to 'invest in' and 'build on' care provi-sion for the future event of childbirth and subsequent motherhood. The disappointment they reported if they had not been present at the birth reflected the personal satisfaction this investment could give them. Comments made at such times were particularly illuminating:

> You are with them for all that time and then miss out at the end – you've missed the bloody party! That's what I feel.   (Caseload midwife 18)

> It's like revising for an examination and then missing the result. You have put all the hard work in . . . and then you don't know if what you have done has been appropriate.   (Caseload midwife 34)

Caseload practice entailed the midwives becoming more deeply involved with their work than conventional midwifery practice permitted. Such form of engagement could go beyond an 'investment' of their professional skills to ensure a meaningful outcome. It also encompassed something of their individuality that they gave and something that they received in return. The midwives valued the reciprocal relationships established, experiencing enjoyment in the communication and receiving acknowledgement of their personal interests. They valued occasions when their individuality was consid-ered, for example the coffee specially prepared for their visit, or the chats. And they talked of mothers who delayed phoning them because they were aware of some activity in the midwife's personal life, or 'waited' to go into labour until the midwife returned from a weekend off or from holiday.

On a deeper level, the midwives appeared to gain some sense of approbation of their work and being, of why they were a midwife. In defining it as 'real midwifery', they were affirming what they believed midwifery to be, and in being able to practise it in a way that made sense to them, they were able to achieve a sense of self-actualisation (Herzberg et al. 1967; Maslow 1970). No longer acting as the 'caring robots' of conventional service, caseload midwives clearly valued the opportunity to express themselves through their work:

> . . . doing a job that matters. Making a difference by *your* decisions, not just carrying out care that someone else tells you.   (Caseload midwife 20)

> You can portray your life and your personality in your work. (Caseload midwife 16)

For them, the organisational features of caseload midwifery facilitated a realisation of themselves in their work, a situation they had not found possible when working in the conventional services.

Social support

Their relationship also provided an important practical and emotional aspect of social support for both the women and the midwives, something which conventional midwifery care did not appear to facilitate:

> I was just having a horrible time and I just didn't feel there was anybody there for me to talk to. I literally just didn't know what was going on and I went to my classes but it's that emotional side, there was no support at all. I didn't know what I was doing, I just learnt and I still don't even believe I am a mum. Do you know what I mean? That care could have made that little bit of difference. (Conventional care 370)

In contrast, the caseload midwives were able to plan their work to provide more social support to those who needed it most:

> The midwife came to my home to give me the injection. I was very worried at this time as my husband was [in home country] . . . she gave me nice words, reassuring, it was very important, she was friendly and didn't want to rush you.   (Caseload care 48 – refugee separated from husband by visa problems in a 'high risk' multiple pregnancy)

Adjusting to a different style of practice, the midwives soon developed boundaries that clarified the limits of the support they should provide. This discouraged the potential to encourage dependency – the need to be needed – or to encourage women to look to them for all their support, which could also prove unsustainable for the midwife, rather than to facilitate them in finding the other sources of support they needed.

The midwives also developed strong networks of peer support through the partnerships and group practices, something not experienced in conventional practice. Some of the midwives noted how they had developed lasting friendships with their colleagues. However, the satisfaction gained was not confined to working with friends but, more importantly, with like-minded midwives, forming an enduring feature of the caseload model. Although encompassing a wide diversity of personalities and experiences, the midwives shared a similar ethos of practice:

> It's like going to heaven being with midwives that work the same way, who are enthusiastic. I felt this big cloud has lifted!   (Caseload midwives' focus group)

The development of such a degree of support and caring formed an important feature of caseload practice and denies the perception that caseload midwifery encourages an individualistic and isolated approach to work. Such potential may be present but was identified by the midwives as compromising the sustainability and safety of working this way. Elements of their practice that helped to sustain this included working within the group practice for mutual support and back-up but also conducting peer review and discussing their practice during regular meetings and an annual 'awayday'. Clearly, having 'volunteered' to try working with a caseload meant that some element of shared philosophy was present, but the organisation of the practices helped to develop and maintain this, and to prevent individual midwives working in an isolated, unsupported fashion.

Reassurance, confidence and development

Comments from both women and caseload midwives suggested that this organisation of care facilitates the development of confidence and growth for both parties. For some women, the midwife support they received helped them to grow in confidence through the pregnancy and birth, which can be a crucial time of change and adjustment (McCourt 2006). This was especially the case for the younger mothers and those from socially disadvantaged groups. One young woman, for example, had an unplanned pregnancy in her teens, but the midwife helped her to make her own positive choice about it. She felt that she had personally grown through the experience and was now a confident mother, planning further study:

> . . . reassurement and that, 'cos I was still two minded [about the pregnancy]. It was really nice the way she handled the situation. She kept me going and made me finally decide.   (Caseload care 411)

Another discussed how knowing that she could call her midwife at any time if worried gave her more confidence and made her feel less anxious. Women's confidence in the midwife grew through the pregnancy, helping them to prepare for and then cope with the birth:

> well I could talk to her about anything and say to her everything, that's how much confidence I had in her.   (Caseload care 116)

For the midwives, following through care meant they were able to see the outcomes and assess decisions that were made. Continuity made an important 'feedback loop' for learning and evaluation of care provided, which included a significant safety aspect:

> It makes you appreciate the value of today's activity on tomorrow's care. You can see the results of what you do today. If you miss something in hospital it is not so important [inferring the expectation that someone else will pick it up].   (Caseload midwives' focus group)

One midwife described how the ability to follow up and constantly assess the impact of advice given enabled her to change advice to meet individuals' needs, and that she could learn from this and build confidence in her practice; for example: having observed the subsequent healing of a perineum she had sutured, she noted with confidence, 'I now *know* it will not fall apart!'.

Although caseload midwives initially encountered some difficulties and even hostility from their colleagues working in other parts of the maternity service, as time passed in many instances this changed and more positive attitudes developed, with the midwives feeling more acknowledged and respected. The recognition they gained from medical colleagues was highly valued and proved another source of professional satisfaction:

Recognition for professionalism – I found I got that in the caseload project but not in the hospital . . . the doctors may say 'good on you, that was a good decision'.   (Caseload midwife 8)

Not only were the midwives gaining confidence with their clinical skills, their interpersonal and inter-professional communication skills were honed in a manner not facilitated by the conventional service, where conflicts tended to be ignored rather than resolved. The midwives developed skills to work through rather than avoid any of the disputes that inevitably arose, and to be assertive rather than either confrontational or 'avoidant'; this was recognised by senior staff, both medical and managerial, who described them as having 'matured' and developed in ways not generally noted in those working within the conventional service.

Informed choice, control and autonomy

The women tended to feel more fully informed with 'their own' midwife, and in our wider survey, they showed higher expectations of personal control and ability to make decisions about their birth as well as higher satisfaction with the information they were given (Beake et al. 2001). In contrast, women in conventional care, particularly in the hospital setting where care was highly fragmented, often described situations in which lack of information or being given 'empty' information failed to provide the reassurance they needed:

I think that mothers have the right to ask questions and get proper answers and the doctors and nurses need to have more patience with the member of the public really.   (Conventional care 312 – when asked what could be improved about care)

Instead, they often attempted to gain information indirectly, for example by 'reading' professionals' faces, or reading the monitor.

Being informed and feeling they had some control and say in what happened to them was important to how the women felt about their experience, whether they had a straightforward or complicated pregnancy and birth, and appeared to reduce fears and anxieties, whereas lack of information could compound them. This was recognised by the midwives, who commented on how their prior knowledge and discussions with the woman influenced the way they could support them:

You discuss so much before they actually go into labour that when they're in labour it makes it far more easy and you can discuss things better, e.g. fetal monitors. It's all been discussed and then they can see all your reasons why you would do it, why you wouldn't do it. They just come in and they do so much better. Even when they end up with a Caesarean section or whatever they seem to do better afterwards – seem to recover better and psychologically they're better. (Caseload midwife 23)

In assuming a sense of responsibility for their women, and with a greater understanding of an individual's situation, the midwives became more flexible in applying the unit's guidelines concerning labour. Providing they could justify their care plan to the obstetrician's satisfaction, if questioned, the midwives' decisions were usually respected. Where they were not, usually by a less confident registrar who did not know the caseload midwife and imposed intervention routinely, the midwives reported later proactively following up such unsatisfactory management with the delivery unit consultant. In becoming confident to practise and to question medical behaviour in an evidence-based way, the midwives had to be very sure of their own management. This also reflected a growing confidence with their body of midwifery knowledge:

Caseload practice keeps you up there [on top of things], you don't have time to vegetate. If anything came up that you didn't understand you immediately looked it up.   (Caseload midwife 8)

The caseload midwives saw care provision within the conventional service as being limited, in terms of responsibility and decision making, by the lack of continuity:

In the hospital setting if there is something that you're not sure about you pass the buck to either the doctor or whoever's around and often, because you are so busy in the hospital setting, you don't get the chance to follow through to see the outcome, to have it properly explained to you. You pass the buck. Full stop. You've done your responsibility. You've handed it over and you get on with something else; whereas with a caseload it doesn't stop. You have to follow it through. You have to make those decisions and you have to find out for yourself.   (Caseload midwife 6)

The midwives did, nonetheless, learn the value of working with others – when it is appropriate to refer or seek advice – but this did not imply a simple handing over of responsibility, so much as a sharing, since they maintained their role and contact, even when complications arose.

The caseload midwives also described ways in which they could exercise choice and the degree to which autonomy made the system of care and the personal flexibility it demanded possible for them. The midwives managed their own caseloads in partnerships within the group practices. They worked out their own arrangements for providing cover to women, without fixed requirements to work in a particular way. They were primarily answerable to their employers via their caseload. Similarly, they were expected to account for what they did rather than for their time or presence, such as by completing timesheets or clocking in for shifts. It was the unpredictability of birth and women's needs rather than the demands of shifts or rotas that created challenges for them. This was an important feature, since lack of control over their work pattern, such as team midwives being expected to cover for staff shortages on labour wards while maintaining care for a caseload of women, has been highlighted as a major problem in some studies (Green et al. 1998; McCourt et al. 2006).

Holistic and flexible care

It was clear that care provision within the caseload model was more individualised for both women and midwives, meeting their emotional needs and expectations in a more holistic and flexible way than experienced within the conventional service. The hospital setting was seen as being impersonal and rushed, 'like a cattle market', with long waits for hurried visits that were routinised rather than responsive to the women's needs. This environment, stressful for midwives too, often had a negative impact on the care they could provide:

> . . . she worried me unintentionally and she was abrupt. She didn't have any time for me, there was obviously too many people there. (Conventional care 370)

The women described valuing care that paid attention to both their medical *and* their social or psychological needs. They spoke about being understood, being 'cared about' as well as 'cared for' and caseload midwives paying attention to their ordinary needs:

. . . you have no fears or anything you can say to them, look there is something bothering me, how small it is. They don't make you feel as if you are wasting their time.   (Caseload care 116)

In the hospital they found it difficult to ask for or obtain such help. Women with medical problems or complications tended to praise the high standard of medical care they had been given but they described the lack of midwifery input and care for their ordinary needs. For example, following a previous stillbirth one woman reported excellent medical care throughout the birth but felt that her emotional needs were entirely forgotten and her difficulties overlooked once this baby had been born alive; another recognised the good medical care received during an emergency Caesarean but felt entirely abandoned in the post-natal ward. In contrast, 'high risk' women who had a caseload midwife were not transferred from one form of care to another – their midwife maintained the midwifery role, working with the consultant and other professionals as needed, to ensure all-round care was provided.

The midwives particularly valued being able to combine clinical and psychosocial care and saw this as facilitating appropriate care for individual women across this boundary. They discussed their initial fears and then their growing confidence in what they saw as holistic care and using all the skills of midwifery. This included care for women at all levels or types of risk, both medical and psychosocial care and care for all stages and aspects of pregnancy, childbirth and early parenthood. They described this as an important source of personal and professional satisfaction, and associated it with their own, tacit, concept of 'real' midwifery:

You feel you are a midwife – after a while of working this way there will be very little that you don't know about'.   (Caseload midwives' focus group)

The majority of this care was provided at a time that suited both mother and midwife; practising autonomously meant the caseload midwives were completely flexible, working as and when they found appropriate. Thus they could both 'make the job work for them' and work within women's individual time constraints, arranging their schedules in a manner that suited themselves and their partners. The midwives did not have total control over their time as they had to be available to respond to the needs of their women. Nevertheless, once they had developed their personal time management skills and learnt to advise women appropriately, they reported that interruptions at night were minimal and usually confined to labour and emergencies:

> At night? It's not very often. I would say on average a month I would get three. You can't put [a number on it]. Or you may be contacted three times in one night!   (Caseload midwife 6)

Such reporting was verified in a study of caseload midwives' work diaries (McCourt 1998). Knowing the women who contacted them enabled the midwives to respond appropriately, not necessarily having to visit or ask the women to attend hospital but giving advice or making an appointment for the following day. Similarly, the women were reported as not wanting to disturb their midwife unless it was urgent. This symbiotic relationship was seen as an enduring feature of caseload practice, where care and concern was reciprocated and the emotional needs of both women and midwives could be fulfilled.

Conclusions: Should woman-centred care mean midwife unfriendly care?

> I felt this went beyond a job. I felt that she enjoyed her job. Some people that do it . . . don't actually enjoy it, that comes across; but she was so caring.   (Caseload care 391 – about 'her' midwife)

The above quote captures what some women felt about the care provided by caseload midwives, but it also captures some of the concerns and debates aired among midwives about different models of practice. A major question and concern has been whether 'caring work', particularly when offering continuity of carer, is a source of stress and burnout to midwives, making this form of practice ultimately unsustainable for all but an exceptional or dedicated minority. Caring work is clearly demanding, and the woman's comment is suggestive that dedicated midwives may go 'beyond' their job, perhaps beyond what is reasonably demanded of them. However, the picture that emerged from these linked studies gives a very different perspective on the demands and the emotional labour of midwifery work.

Core themes that were identified from the work included aspects of social relationship such as knowing and being known, reciprocity, knowledge and confidence (in self and others). We argue that this model of midwifery care facilitated emotional support for women, and did so without creating additional emotional labour for midwives. Caseload midwives gained satisfaction and reward from their relationships with women. A high level of autonomy in their practice, and the ability to form supportive relationships with women and with colleagues was important to their ability to cope well with the demands of their role. Nevertheless this could easily and often be undermined by tensions with colleagues working in different models of care and in the interface with the service-providing institution.

It was clear from the women's narratives that they viewed the care given in the caseload system as more woman-centred (or indeed family-centred). This applied particularly to women who were socially disadvantaged, young or from minority ethnic groups. Was this provided at the expense of woman-centred work for midwives, conforming to a caring ideal that makes unreasonable demands on their time and energy? The evidence we gathered did not support this conclusion. The flexibility required of the midwives to provide continuity of carer was also balanced by the greater control they experienced over their patterns of work, allowing them to gain some flexibility in their lives. A key sustainability issue, alongside that of relationship and reciprocity, was the level of autonomy this organisation of practice facilitated.

The midwives described their own development in terms of confidence and decision making. This included greater confidence in making clinical judgements, greater confidence and assertiveness in referring women when they felt more specialist advice or care was needed, and greater confidence in working outside the hospital. The midwives were required (and learned) to be highly self-managing in terms of time, management of their caseload and workload, defining appropriate boundaries and their place of work but were also able to work effectively with their peers. These changes were underpinned by greater autonomy, decision making and locus of responsibility and control. However, the structural position of midwives had not changed to facilitate this, as reflected in the many tensions the midwives encountered at interfaces between different parts of the service.

Caseload midwives were able to achieve a sense of self-actualisation that they had not found in the conventional service, as exemplified in the movement from 'role' of midwife to 'being' a midwife; this was an important constituent of the job satisfaction they expressed. It has been suggested that workers not fulfilling such a need could result in a sense of alienation, disconnection and associated loss of meaning about their work (Herzberg et al. 1967). Marxist notions of alienation hold strong resonance with conventional maternity services – involving a separation of worker from the product of their labour, a fragmentation of the work process so it becomes task orientated and eventually meaningless, and domination by market forces rather than relationships (Martin 1987; Robinson 1990). It might also explain the concern raised by Jean Robinson of AIMS (Association for Improvements in the Maternity Services) (Robinson 2000: 143) who, following receipt of a number of complaints from mothers, questioned: 'Why are midwives turning nasty?' The relationship, once the fulcrum of a midwife's work, now holds minimal significance to midwives working in conventional services.

The findings of our research suggest that caseload midwifery, if it is supported by appropriate structural and organisational changes, can redress this imbalance. This is achieved through the development of a reciprocal relationship that the prolonged contact facilitates. Mothers have the opportunity to address any sense of indebtedness they may feel towards the care provider, the midwife, enhancing their sense of control. Perhaps more significantly, midwives benefit from the reciprocal relationship by its contribution towards high levels of job satisfaction and less stress, thus reducing the potential for 'burnout'. These midwives gained great satisfaction and a sense of reward from their relationships with the women, something which sustained their practice and may provide a key to its sustainability.

Reflective questions

1   Given the findings of our research detailed in this chapter, how far do you consider it is possible that the ability to offer continuity of carer can benefit midwives even more than women? In what ways may this occur?

2   In providing continuity of care the caseload midwives highlighted how this enabled them to learn from 'their' women. How do you learn from the women you care for? How might this be influenced by the organisation of midwifery services in your area and how might it differ from caseload practice?

3   The relationships that caseload midwives were able to form with their women proved important for their own emotional well-being and was central to the sustainability of this model of practice. In your practice what do you find to be most stressful and what factors help to maintain your motivation?

References

Beake, S., McCourt, C. and Page, L. eds (2001) *Evaluation of One-to-One Midwifery: Second Cohort Study* (London: Thames Valley University).

Deery, R. (2005) An action research study exploring midwives' support needs and the effect of group clinical supervision, *Midwifery,* 21: 161–76.

Department of Health (1993) *Changing Childbirth: Report of the Expert Maternity Group* (London: HMSO).

Green, J., Curtis, P., Price, H. and Renfrew, M. (1998) *Continuing to Care: The Organization of Midwifery Dervices in the UK: A Structured Review of the Evidence* (Cheshire: Books for Midwives Press).

Herzberg, F., Mausner, B. and Snyderman, B. (1967) *The Motivation to Work* (New York: John Wiley).

Hunter, B. (2004) Conflicting ideologies as a source of emotion work in midwifery, *Midwifery,* 20(3): 261–72.

Kirkham, M. (1989) Midwives and information giving during labour. In: S. Robinson and A. Thomson (eds), *Midwives, Research and Childbirth,* Volume I (London: Chapman & Hall).

Martin, E. (1987) *The Woman in the Body: A Cultural Analysis of Reproduction* (Boston, MA: Beacon Press).

Maslow, A. (1970) *Motivation and Personality* (Harlow: Longman).

McCourt, C. (1998) Working patterns of caseload midwives: a diary analysis, *British Journal of Midwifery,* 6(9): 580–5.

McCourt, C. (2006) Becoming a parent. In: L. Page and R. McCandlish (eds), *The New Midwifery: Science and Sensitivity in Practice,* 2nd edn (Oxford: Churchill Livingstone).

McCourt, C., Stevens, T., Sandall, J. and Brodie, P. (2006) Working with women: continuity of carer in practice. In: L. Page and R. McCandlish (eds), *The New Midwifery: Science and Sensitivity in Practice,* 2nd edn (Oxford: Churchill Livingstone).

Methven, R. (1989) Recording an obstetric history or relating to pregnant women? A study of the antenatal booking interview. In: S. Robinson and A. M. Thomson (eds), *Midwives, Research and Childbirth,* Volume 1 (London: Chapman & Hall).

Robinson, J. (2000) Why are midwives turning nasty? *British Journal of Midwifery,* 8(2): 143.

Robinson, S. (1990) Maintaining the independence of the midwifery profession: a continuing struggle. In: J. Garcia, R. Kilpatrick and M. Richards (eds), *The Politics of Maternity Care* (Oxford: Oxford University Press).

Sandall, J. (1997) Midwives' burnout and continuity of care, *British Journal of Midwifery,* 5(2): 106–11.

Stevens T. (2003) Midwife to midwif: a study of caseload midwifery. PhD thesis, London, Thames Valley University.

Stevens, T. and McCourt, C. (2001) One-to-one midwifery practice – part 1: setting the scene, *British Journal of Midwifery,* 9(12): 736–40.

Stevens, T. and McCourt, C. (2002a) One-to-one midwifery practice – part 2: the transition period, *British Journal of Midwifery*, 10(1): 45–50.

Stevens, T. and McCourt, C. (2002b) One-to-one midwifery practice – part 3: meaning for midwives, *British Journal of Midwifery*, 10(2): 111–15.

Stevens, T. and McCourt, C. (2002c) One-to-one midwifery practice – part 4: sustaining the model, *British Journal of Midwifery*, 10(3): 174–9.

2

Women's Emotion Work in the Context of Current Maternity Services

Nadine Pilley Edwards

Introduction

In this chapter, I explore the notion that women, like midwives, are doing emotion work and that it can be equally damaging or rewarding for both groups. I use the terms 'emotional work', 'emotional labour' and 'emotion work' cautiously, to acknowledge that they are not necessarily interchangeable. McClure and Murphy (2007) suggest that we need more nuanced definitions of different facets of emotion management, which reflect that which is done in a paid/use context (emotional labour), that which is unpaid/exchange (emotion work), and that which usually takes place in the work situation, but which is unrecognised and unpaid, and might include both use and exchange values (emotional work). This will be exceedingly complex to define, particularly for midwives and women engaging across the public/private and paid/unpaid boundaries, which are themselves constructed within a health provision context where the notion of 'consumer' and 'consumerism' has become a central point of reference. Meantime, I have referred to the emotional labour of midwives, the emotion work of women and emotional work when talking collectively about midwives and women. I discuss how emotion work is entangled with entrenched societal values and beliefs which set a trajectory for the complex processes of medicalisation and consumerism. These processes have developed and maintained a philosophy of birth care, birth practices and social structures that place many constraints on both women and midwives, distance them from themselves and each other, and cause dissonance that is harmful to their well-being. This has devastating consequences not only for the individual woman, family and midwife, but also for attempts to work together. Transforming emotional work into a resource amidst such complexities requires us to simultaneously illuminate the wider issues in society that underlie the muting and devaluing of emotional work, make more visible the ensuing oppressive processes which cause it to be damaging, and build on initiatives that support collective, emotional well-being.

We have a developing tapestry of what emotional work entails, and how it affects both the private and public spheres of our lives. We have more recently gained insights into how midwives perceive and 'do' emotional labour. We have a growing body of literature that tells us about the positive and negative emotional impacts of birth, and of health practitioners and other support people on women. The missing pieces are to do with what kind of emotion work women are carrying out in relation to their experiences of birth, birth practices, attendants and services, and the effects this has on them.

Emotional labour, emotion work and emotional work are more closely defined in the introduction to this book. For the purposes of this chapter, I draw attention to two key points. The first centres on the use of emotion for commercial gain (Hochschild 1983). Emotions and emotional work have had strong links with capitalism. Karl Marx himself described the worker's alienation from paid work as a central outcome of capitalism and the manipulation of emotions was seen as a profitable monetary resource (Caffrey 2007). The commercial use of emotional labour is growing in the health service industry, where efficient processing of the 'customer' is paramount (Bolton 2002; Bone 2002). This, along with the processes of industrialisation, greatly affects maternity services and the emotional work of midwives and women.

The second point is that emotional work is a feature of all human relationships both within and outside the workplace. As we know from the introduction, and other literature, emotional labour is about 'dealing with other people's emotions' (James 1989: 15) in a variety of ways (Calhoun 1992 in Frith and Kitzinger 1998: 118; McClure and Murphy 2007), often at a 'cost to the worker' (Hunter 2001: 437) who must maintain a 'professional demeanour' (Earle et al. 2007: 27). It is seen as both a positive resource (Hochschild 1983; Bolton 2000; McCreight 2005; Hunter 2006) and as a negative, oppressive expectation of the predominantly female caring professions (James 1992; Bolton 2000; Deery 2003; Deery and Kirkham 2007). It has been similarly defined as a resource, or oppressive in familial and social networks (Higgins and

Werner-Wilson 1997; Frith and Kitzinger 1998). The complex relationship between the paid, professional midwife, and the women performing the intimate act of birth has been examined in many different ways, but in terms of any theorised notion about the emotion work that women do in relation to birth attendants and maternity services, there is complete silence. Yet, in my study about women's experiences of planning home births (Edwards 2001, 2005), women talk in the same terms as those described in the literature about midwives.

The impact of midwives' emotional labour on women

We can see that childbirth is emotional, and that women have both profoundly positive, life-enhancing experiences and deeply traumatic experiences, and that supportive care during childbearing has a major impact on these experiences (Kirkham 2000; Robinson 2004; Kitzinger 2006; McCourt et al. 2006). Even quantitative work, which cannot easily identify qualitative aspects of birth, suggests that this is so: 'supportive care may have long-term effects and may protect some women from a long-term negative experience' (Waldenstrom 2004: 17), and 'of the established methods to improve women's birth experiences . . . support in labour and listening to women's own issues may be underestimated' (Waldenstrom et al. 2004: 102).

We can see how the way midwives manage their emotions has an impact on women. For example, midwives often report that midwifing is 'stressful, but I'm one of those people who can be quite stressed inside but calm on the outside . . .', and 'I've seemed as cool as a cucumber . . . yet my insides feel like a food mixer . . .' (John and Parsons 2006: 268). A woman in my study (Edwards 2001) reported how beneficial the midwife's being 'as cool as a cucumber' was when she had a long labour that she struggled with:

> obviously it was my decision as to how much I could take but in the end it was all fine . . . But I mean basically, you know she [midwife] stayed as cool as a cucumber, which you know, if she hadn't, if she'd at any point suggested that I wasn't going to make it then that would have had a huge influence on me, you know, 'cos I would have said, 'oh, great you agree. Okay, I can't do it.'   (Edwards 2001: 240)

From the work carried out by Mavis Kirkham and Ruth Deery (Kirkham 1999; Deery 2003; Kirkham and Stapleton 2004; Deery and

Kirkham 2006, 2007), we can imagine the stressful emotional labour that must have been taken on by a community midwife who supported a woman's need to avoid vaginal examinations in labour, against the needs of a midwifery colleague to do them, and then to continue to support the woman to stay at home for the birth of her placenta that took over four hours, despite requests from the hospital to transfer the woman immediately:

> I was really glad that [midwife] was there. Afterwards I was crying when I thought of what could have happened if we had had another midwife. I just kept saying 'thanks be to god, thanks be to god' all the way through 'cos I would have been in hospital. She was a great support and it could have been very different, you know.   (Edwards 2005: 225)

We can also see the regulatory, coercive aspects of emotional labour as it is played out by health practitioners: for example, when they evoke feelings of fear, uncertainty, selfishness, guilt, blame, irrationality and even silliness, or threaten withdrawal, to make sure women behave 'appropriately' – that is, in line with local policies and practices. For example, a woman decided to give birth to her placenta physiologically, without the use of Syntometrine, but her midwives and GP were very against this. When I first interviewed her, she told me that 'if everything goes the way I'm hoping and everything's natural then I'm just going to carry on. I don't see why I should get some intervention, when everything's going so fine'. Later in her pregnancy, during a second interview, she told me that she had been persuaded to accept Syntometrine, and that not only had she 'given in', but that she was not 'going to be silly about it' (Edwards 2001: 221–2). Another woman, who was considered 'high risk', was asked how the rest of her family would feel if her baby was brain damaged during birth (Edwards 2005: 105). Thus, being defined as a good mother is apparently dependent on accepting questionable obstetric ideology (Murphy-Lawless 1998; Edwards and Murphy-Lawless 2006).

Women's emotion work

So the hard graft of midwives' emotional labour (to 'convey the right emotions for each situation', act as if 'delighted with every birth', 'behave as if instrumental deliveries were not horrific events' and show pleasure not boredom when with a woman having an epidural) is reported as draining and stressful, 'more challenging than . . . antici-pated' (Earle et al. 2007: 27), but a 'necessary part of the job' (John and Parsons 2006: 268). This work, which can create a kind of cognitive dissonance for many midwives, can be supportive, or constraining, for women. But emotional work is not something only midwives do. We can see that emotion work is implicit in much of the feminist literature on agency, decision making and relationships (Gilligan 1985; Belenky et al. 1986; Debold et al. 1996). For example:

> Even when women held strongly to their own ways of doing things, they remained concerned about not hurting the feelings of their opponents by openly expressing dissent. They reported that they were apt to hide their opinions and then suffer quietly the frustration of not standing up to others. Some women described feeling either petulant, private resentment of others or self-admonishment for being so unassertive.   (Belenky et al. 1986: 84)

While there are conflicting views in this area of work, typically, women tend not to assert their needs, if this might jeopardise relation-ships. This is very much the case in midwifery and birth (Murphy-Lawless 1998; Smythe 1998; Anderson 2000; Edwards 2004; Deery and Kirkham 2006). For example, midwives have largely accepted a culture of 'service and sacrifice', where they look after others, but feel it is 'self-ish' to address personal needs (Deery and Kirkham 2006: 125), and women also reluctantly compromise or feel guilty about not complying with others. So just as midwives are reluctant to 'rock the boat' (Hunter and Deery 2005: 12), so are women. For example, one woman 'agreed' to a scan she did not believe was necessary or safe, because, 'if I contest the scan, maybe she [GP] won't be so supportive of me. I better do this to show that I am willing to co-operate and I didn't want to make waves' (Edwards 2001: 249); and another woman reported sadly that, 'I can feel quite strongly about what I want, and I can go for it to a certain extent and then there's a point at which it becomes too difficult for me' (Edwards 2001: 250).

When, very occasionally, a woman did openly assert herself, she worried about alienating midwives, and about her decision-making abilities:

> the more angry and adamant she [midwife] got, the more adamant I got that this [home birth] was my choice. But it's when you get

home that you start to think, god what a big head to head I've had there and these are the women that are supposed to be coming and giving me care and if I alienate them I won't get the best care. Or perhaps I have made a bit of a silly choice . . . you end up with self doubt – whether you are making the right decision.   (Edwards 2005: 221–2)

From the negative experiences of birth described in some of the birth trauma literature (Kitzinger 1992; Kitzinger 2006; AIMS 2007), we can assume that women are obliged to engage in a high level of emotion work, as they struggle to appear to be coping, care for their babies, and function well as family members and workers, while feeling depressed, shocked, violated and traumatised:

I wanted to rewind the tape. . . . As I left the hospital five days later after this event [birth], I felt my life was in pieces.   (Quipp-Stenson 2007: 15)

We can see that this work might continue for many years, as they continue to experience feelings that contradict the accepted 'feeling rules' (Hochschild 1983) of joy and happiness around birth:

I should have been able to receive this news [of a niece being born] with pure joy, but I am finding it impossible to access that joy through the tears and anguish that I have been left with through my own births . . . My sons' births were hideous . . . I want to scream out for what should have been . . . these effects last a lifetime, this is not something I will get over, this is something that will continue to come back and haunt me.   (Chippington-Derrick 2007: 8)

These reported experiences immediately plunge us into the complexities of emotional work: the work of managing immediate and ongoing emotions in the self and others, in the context of negotiating deeply held ideological and social norms around birthing and motherhood. Women's emotion work is therefore about resistance and compliance, identity and agency. Part of this debate is thus about examining this emotional work, in order to make the oppressive and damaging ideologies and practices around birth and elsewhere more visible, and so perhaps transform them.

Why is emotion work relatively invisible?

The concept of emotion work and labour and their uncertain practices lie within a web of technological and capitalist imperatives (Murphy-Lawless 2006; Pollock 2006), and behind that web lies a wash of patriarchal notions of rationality (Colebrook 1997; Murphy-Lawless 1998; Edwards 2005; McCreight 2005). The impact of these on the distribution, visibility and value of emotion work and emotional labour is that not only are women expected to do most of it, but it is defined as unproductive work and remains largely 'undefined, unexplained and usually unrecorded' (Bolton 2000: 581). Consequently, it is not well taught, to nurses or to midwives (Smith 1991; James 1992; McQueen 2004; McCreight 2005), because women are assumed to know what to do, and get on with it, no matter what (James 1992: 501). Thus, in a *Panorama* programme (BBC1, 3 May 2007) on midwifery shortages, when a stressed midwife lets her guard slip, suggesting that a woman in labour 'get a life', we are shocked.

Not only is emotion work and emotional labour muted, but in health care, the technological thinking bound up with contemporary capitalist practices creates increasingly industrial, task-orientated practices that claim to contain, manage and fix bodies as efficiently as possible, rather than focus on ways of relating to sentient beings. Bodies are seen as mechanistic rather than a complex body–mind dialogue that practitioners need to listen to and engage with. Indeed, research suggests that training in health care involves socialisation away from caring qualities and attitudes (Carkhuff 1984; Davis Floyd and St John 1998). Thus, the empirical reality of 'doing' tasks rather than feeling or being with hides behind the professional rhetoric of caring (Smith 1991: 75). Emotions are on the whole seen as distractions, so emotional labour must be fitted in, in addition to the real work: 'Having been sitting talking to a patient a nurse would say "I must do some work now", meaning it was time to do some physical tasks' (James 1992: 497).

This technological orientation has devastating impacts on individuals, groups and indeed on nations. The poorer and more oppressed, the more devastating are the consequences. A chilling example is provided by Barbara Ehrenreich's and Arlie Hochschild's (2002) moving book, *Global Woman*. This shows the 'toxicity' (Deery 2003) of emotion work in contemporary society (work that is mostly done by poor women and children) when love and care are commodified to service wealthy nations.

The impact of ideology on emotion work

So, birthing women are obliged to deal with their own emotions in relation to obstetric definitions of appropriate birth practices and appropriate behaviour. They have to deal with the disruption to relationships
caused by these beliefs and practices, that are so deeply held, and which
they question. They must manage themselves and their emotions, to be
seen to be responsible, intelligent and reasonable in order to negotiate
with health carers and at the same time protect themselves and their
babies. They are obliged to deal, somehow, with the overt and covert
attacks on their identities as 'proper' pregnant women with credible
knowledge and experience.

In the same way that Billie Hunter (2004) identified conflicting
ideologies to be at the heart of the emotional labour and work of
midwives, I found this to be at the heart of the emotion work of women
planning home births (Edwards 2005, 2001). Hunter found that the
untenable position of midwives between midwifery practice, medical
policies, employers and women (Murphy-Lawless 1991; Clarke 1995;
Levy 1999; Hunter 2000; Kirkham and Stapleton 2001) was greatly
reduced in the community. Women planning home births agreed that
avoiding large obstetric units offers some protection from the coercive
pull of medicalisation (Machin and Scamell 1997), but they pointed out
that they were still subjected to the same ideology, albeit from more of
a distance (Edwards 2005).

Pregnant women want birth to be as straightforward and least trau-
matising as possible. Achieving this might mean a home birth for one
woman, and an elective Caesarean for another, though most women do
not want interventions and research suggests that less intervention is
associated with greater satisfaction (Green et al. 1998). But the focus on
reducing interventions and increasing midwifery care in the community has to be painstakingly negotiated. The challenge for women is to
remain calm and reasonable as they negotiate their deeply held views of
what is best, with the obstetric view of what is best, *and*, among the
compromises, retain some autonomy and integrity. This mirrors
Hochschild's claim that the worker's problem is, 'how to adjust one's
self to the role in a way that allows some self in the role but minimizes
the stress the role puts on the self' (Staden 1998: 154). However they
managed this, just like health practitioners, most felt some degree of
discomfort, distress, fear, anxiety and distrust (see Strange 2002;
McCreight 2005; McClure and Murphy 2007).

Disengaging: distancing rather than 'being with'

In the current context of staff shortages, high workloads, lack of educational input, fragmented care, lack of time and lack of support, numbers of studies in midwifery report that stress and burnout is common (Sandall 1997; Hunter 2001; Ball et al. 2002; Deery and Kirkham 2007) and that task orientation follows. Using Mary Douglas's (1966) concept of 'matter out of place', Ruth Deery and Mavis Kirkham suggest that: 'In a large-scale, industrial model of maternity care, distressing emotions can only be experienced as matter which is out of place, impeding the smooth running of the "conveyor belt" of the service' (Deery and Kirkham 2007: 81).

In the context of fragmented relationships, women tend to take their cues from midwives. Thus if midwives keep to the tasks in hand, keep their 'emotional lids' on, and fear 'leaking feelings' as a sign of lack of control (Deery and Kirkham 2006: 134), women do the same. So while women felt that care should be more than physical checks, they found that short visits with faceless practitioners made it impossible to discuss more intimate, emotional aspects of birth. Emotional matters become 'matter out of place' for them too. So, although one woman felt that it was crucial for midwives to know about her fears and strengths:

> I could bet my bottom dollar that there was no question that would ever address that. And I couldn't ask questions like that because it would be so jarring. It would just be so personal. It would be like I was gushing all over them if I'd said anything like, I need to discuss how I feel about being naked in front of a complete stranger, or I need to discuss how I feel about making noises. It would seem embarrassing. I'm not embarrassed to discuss these things but in the framework of the NHS system it would be very embarrassing to bring that up. You know within that setting to try and bring up more emotional complex issues would feel quite wrong. You would feel like you crossed the boundary.   (Edwards 2001: 223–4)

Just as women find it an effort to engage with midwives, midwives report that women 'drain you', '[wring] every ounce out of you', and '[absorb] every bit of energy' (Deery and Kirkham 2007: 74). In order to cope, they create boundaries, and stereotype women to discount the needs they cannot meet (p. 78). Unable to find any other way of processing emotional labour, they distance themselves from each other and from women. Disengaging becomes another habitual coping strategy for health practitioners (Greenhall 2001: 112; Hunter 2001; Hunter and Deery 2005). Women experience this detachment as 'formulaic':

> They [midwives] were very helpful, but one thing I would say is that they seem to have been trained how to treat people and the sorts of problems people have and the sorts of anxieties people have. And when they're faced with you, you're an individual . . . and I didn't sometimes think that I was being heard . . . and, do you know, I didn't feel there was a dialogue. I felt a little bit invisible. It was a bit smiley and a bit formulaic.   (Edwards 2005: 174)

Many women responded to this lack of engagement by attempting to breech the insurmountable barriers of conflicting ideologies, lack of time and lack of continuity, and appreciated attempts by practitioners to do the same. But some described practitioners as 'jaded', and became 'jaded' themselves. They talked about 'that division between you, and I don't know whether it can be crossed really', others about 'relying on my partner', 'not putting too much emphasis on the midwife', seeing her 'as somebody there to deal with emergencies and do the paperwork' (Edwards 2005: 181; Edwards 2001: 238).

So while Billie Hunter (2001: 438) suggests that emotional exhaustion (burnout) and the resulting disengagement among midwives largely results from industrialised services that leave them unable to 'do' emotional labour, these services had a similar impact on the women I interviewed (Edwards 2001, 2005). They also felt unable to 'do' the emotion work of negotiating across ideologies with individual midwives and eventually some gave up on relationships. The sheer effort of trying to engage with midwives in these contexts was overwhelming, sometimes upsetting, if not impossible; even with teams of six to eight midwives (and 'teams' may now include between 15 and 20 midwives), 'you never really scratch the surface', 'you can't knock six of them into shape by meeting them all once each', and

> even if you manage to reach an understanding with one of them, you don't know if they're going to be there and it's quite exhausting in fact to have to make that effort six times over.   (Edwards 2005: 199)

The combination of midwives distancing themselves behind tasks and policies led women to feel that they could not trust midwives to support their birthing intentions, or protect them, and to feel that they too must hide their feelings:

> I just thought that every time I conveyed a fear, it was going to be another black mark against me being able to stay at home or something so I began to develop a habit of hiding things. I just answered her [midwife] questions in a very bland way.   (Edwards 2001: 229)

Sometimes, even though they needed support, some women felt the stresses on midwives were such that while they thought that the midwife's role was to increase confidence in them, they felt obliged to manage their own doubts and reassure their midwives:

> I always feel they should be more confident and they should make me not have any doubts myself. But I always feel I end up trying to encourage them to think it's going to be alright.   (Edwards 2005: 113)

In other words, like midwives, women hide emotional distress, and put on their 'masks' (Hunter 2000: 34) for the outside world, appearing calm on the outside, while feeling stressed inside, in order to present and evoke the 'right' emotions.

The constraints on midwives to practise midwifery and the resulting disengagement undermines women's decisions, if they fear that they might be 'persuaded' into agreeing to procedures that they did not want at a 'vulnerable moment'. This anxiety was often contained and transformed into a vague or forlorn 'hoping for the best' without any basis for this. One can hear the utter relief when women find midwives who can engage with them supportively. They can let go of all the intricate, exhausting and worrying negotiations:

> the difference of knowing I'd have someone more in line with my thinking – I didn't feel that I needed a birth plan any more. I don't need all these things because I trust her opinion and that way I don't have any fears. So I don't have to swot up so much and be so defensive.   (Edwards 2001: 239)

But because of the constraints on midwives, it was rare to hear about these transformations. Mostly women changed their expectations.

Women's expectations

We know that women are socialised to expect little of maternity care (Green et al. 1998), expect what is on offer (Porter and MacIntyre 1984;

Teijlingen et al. 2003), and submit to medicalised care (Davis-Floyd 1992; Machin and Scamell 1997; Miller 1998). We can perhaps assume that this entails distressing emotion work, but we know little about how this occurs at a deeper level, and how it interacts with the lowering of women's expectations throughout their lives, and how much emotion work has been, and is being, done out of sight, to reconcile women's internal and external worlds (Debold et al. 1996; Hamer 1999).

Just as midwives increasingly let go of their ideals and 'walk away' (Hunter and Deery 2005: 12), so do women. One woman who worked hard to engage her midwives during her first pregnancy described herself this time round as 'much more businesslike. My approach is just, "let them get on with their side of it and I get on with my side"' (Edwards 2005: 219).

Transforming emotional labour and emotion work

While many oppressive factors might impact on women's and midwives' lives, obstetric ideology and the structures, policies and practices it maintains are deeply undermining of women's and midwives' self-esteem and autonomy (Murphy-Lawless 1998; Edwards 2005; Kitzinger 2006; Deery and Kirkham 2007). How do we stop midwives becoming 'burnt out' and blaming themselves and women? How do we ensure that women gain strength and courage from birthing their babies, to set them up on their womanhood/motherhood journeys, so that they feel that, 'if we can do this, we can do anything', rather than feeling sad, violated and traumatised, that they 'should have been stronger', that they 'let [themselves] down', that they lost control of their responsibility to their babies (Edwards 2005: 124, 251,199)?

How can we stop the destructive paradox: that what can be most empowering for women might jeopardise midwives' relationships and employment, and what might be most protective for midwives might necessitate coercing women to compromise on what they believe is best for themselves and their babies? How can we resolve the damaging ironies, that both women and midwives have to work so hard – women to resist routine medical birth, and midwives to enforce it, when birth is essentially a process of letting go (Anderson 2000), and, that maternity services are organised around the erasure of emotion and emotional labour from an emotionally charged event?

What more do we need to do to dispel the myth that continuity, holistic care, and professional friendship is currently being provided, when, 'the concept of working with people's emotional needs is at odds with [the] "technical-rational" paradigm' (Hunter 2001: 438)?

Currently, the overly technocratised and industrialised model of birth leads to increasing amounts of energy being expended to create increasing levels of toxicity for midwives and trauma for women. This does not improve birth outcomes and worsens experiences. Energy would be better spent on promoting social, midwifery models of care that can improve outcomes as well as women's and midwives' experiences.

There are stunning examples of women and midwives working together in ways that Billie Hunter and Trudy Stevens describe as 'reciprocal' (Stevens 2003; Hunter 2006). Other examples (Sandall et al. 2001; Kirkham 2003; Leatherbarrow et al. 2004; Walsh 2007) show that holistic care in smaller settings such as Birth Centres and women's homes, which provide enough continuity to develop trusting relationships, can transform what has become 'toxic' for women and midwives to 'nutrient learning material' which promotes growth (Deery and Kirkham 2007: 81). These ways of working invariably create virtuous cycles where the development of attributes that best support midwives (Deery and Kirkham 2006: 131) – trusting relationships, reciprocity, high degrees of autonomy, and holistic approaches to birth – also best support women.

When this happens, the positive cycles that occur mean that emotional and practical labour can be shared out among midwives, so that they can meet not only women's needs, but each other's, without suffering the consequences of 'toxic' burnout (McCourt et al. 2006; Walsh 2007).

The inclusivity of maternity services and the provision of safe care depend at least partially on emotional work that is mutually supportive for women and practitioners. This requires explicitly educating 'emotionally intelligent practitioners' (McQueen 2004; Hunter and Smith 2007: 860), developing broadly shared values, creating structures that provide time for trusting relationships between women and midwives to grow, and fostering mutual autonomy skills. This would enable the next quotation to become usual rather than unique:

> there was a kind of silence in the relationship, a stillness which was very important. And we'd done all the talking in the build up. So the talking was done. I felt confident that she [midwife] knew where I was coming from and vice versa. It was like we'd done all our dress rehearsal – what if . . . what if . . . And on the day there was nothing left to say really. So it just felt very calm, and I think that was the most important thing.   (Edwards 2005: 180)

Individual midwives have worked ingeniously for years, thwarting the technocratic imperative, with greater or lesser success. For years, women too, have ingeniously engaged their attendants and used every ounce of their skills to assert their autonomy around birthing. Both groups of women have suffered the consequences when their ingenuity and skills have not been enough. The technological imperative, the industrialisation of services (Dykes 2006; Deery and Kirkham 2007) and the resulting 'time bind syndrome' (Hochschild 2003) binds us all in ways that no amount of ingenuity can keep getting around. Unless we can move towards the kind of initiatives above, ingenuity will eventually run out of steam, as we are steamrollered into roles evoking intolerable levels of stress.

Conclusion

Highlighting emotion work and labour is one way of examining the clash between patriarchal, capitalist ideologies that foster massively destructive inequalities, where oppressed groups and individuals are obliged to grapple with material, physical, emotional and spiritual dissonances, and workers feel obliged to accept their own damaging exploitation. Seeing the connections between ideology and health care practices helps us to see how emotional labour and work become burdens when health practitioners accept the role of containing and managing emotion in themselves and their clients so as not to disrupt the 'smooth running of the service' (Deery and Kirkham 2007: 78), a service which is increasingly pared down and privatised as the state reduces its commitment to quality health services (Pollock 2006).

This is not usually about individual practitioners or women; it is not even about obstetrics and midwifery. This is about dominant value systems that value measureable outcomes, not emotional work (James 1992; Greenhall 2001: 112): value systems that greatly reduce possibilities for positive human interactions between health carer and person, by defining productivity and efficiency in terms of objects and tasks, and deploying resources on centralisation and technology rather than on the quality of care and more humane settings. The process of changing the neoliberal[1] health care package is particularly challenging, as it also means changing the neoliberal ordering of the world: a neoliberal order that favours low taxes and reduced public services. Of course there is ambivalence about this, as this regime provides material benefits. Meanwhile, midwives and mothers 'pay a high price for the maintenance of such order' (Deery and Kirkham 2007: 78). Only we can decide when that price is too high and begin to work more collaboratively to critically examine the drivers behind the health care system, and transform this knowledge into transformatory action. Only we can begin to value what has been ignored for very many years: women, babies, families, midwives, relationships, feelings, quality of life – all those aspects that contribute to 'social capital' (Smith 1988; Tones and Green 2002) rather than purely economic capital. We need to break the oppressive, collective silence about emotional work and verbalise the 'collective nature' of all of our experiences (Hunter and Deery 2005: 15) in order to socialise and humanise birth for women, babies, families and midwives.

Reflective questions

1   Can you think of examples of emotional labour that you do that help you to develop as a midwife, and examples of emotional labour that you do that are undermining and stressful for you?

2   How do you think that the emotional labour you do affects the women you care for?

3   Could you make any changes that would reduce the damaging impacts of emotional labour and/or increase its positive impacts for you and women?

Note

1   I use the term neoliberal to refer to the 'deregulation, privatisation, and withdrawal of the state from many areas of social provision' (Harvey 2005: 3). Many aspects of life have been commodified and abandoned to increasingly unregulated market forces which benefit a small number of large corporations. While health care in Britain in the past was somewhat protected from these forces, over the last decades, it has been steadily privatised and profitable areas have been taken over by multinational agencies and corporations, with an almost invariable drop in the quality of services (Pollock 2006).

References

AIMS (2007) Birth Trauma Journal, *AIMS Journal* 19(1). Available from www.aims.org.uk.

Anderson, T. (2000) Feeling safe enough to let go: The relationship between a woman and her midwife during the second stage of labour. In: M. Kirkham (ed.), *The Midwife–Mother Relationship* (Basingstoke: Palgrave Macmillan), pp. 92–119.

Ball, L., Curtis, P. and Kirkham, M. (2002). *Why Do Midwives Leave?* (London: Royal College of Midwives Publications).

Belenky, M. F., Clinchy, B. M., Goldberger, N. R. and Tarule, J. M. (1986) *Women's Ways of Knowing: The Development of Self, Voice and Mind* (New York: Basic Books).

Bolton, S. C. (2000) Who cares? Offering emotion work as a 'gift' in the nursing labour process, *Journal of Advanced Nursing*, 32(3): 580–6.

Bolton S. C. (2002) Consumer as king in the NHS, *International Journal of Public Sector Management*, 15(2): 129–39.

Bone, D. (2002) Dilemmas of emotion work in nursing under market-driven health care, *International Journal of Public Sector Management*, 15(2): 140–50.

Caffrey, B. (2007) Emotion work. In: *Why Work? Sociological Answers* http://www.whywork.org.uk//chapter_6.htm (accessed July 2007)

Carkhuff, R. R. (1984) *Helping and Human Relations*, 2 vols (Amherst, MA: Human Resource Development Press; first published 1969).

Chippington-Derrick, D. (2007) Aftershocks, *AIMS Journal*, 19(1): 8.

Clarke, R. A. (1995) Midwives, their employers and the UKCC: An eternally unethical triangle, *Nursing Ethics*, 2(3): 247–53.

Colebrook, C. (1997) Feminism and autonomy: The crisis of the self-authoring subject, *Body and Society*, 3(2): 21–41.

Davis-Floyd, R. E. (1992) *Birth as an American Rite of Passage* (Berkeley, CA: University of California Press).

Davis-Floyd, R. E, and St John, G., eds (1998) *From Doctor to Healer: The Transformative Journey* (New Brunswick, NJ: Rutgers University Press).

Debold, E., Tolman, D. and Brown, L. M. (1996) Embodying knowledge, knowing desire: Authority and split subjectivities in girls' epistemological development. In: N. Goldberger, J. Tarule, B. Clinchy and M. Belenky (eds), *Knowledge, Difference, and Power: Essays Inspired by Women's Ways of Knowing* (New York: Basic Books), pp. 85–125.

Deery, R. (2003) Engaging with clinical supervision in a community midwifery setting: an action research study. Unpublished PhD thesis, University of Sheffield, UK.

Deery, R. and Kirkham, M. (2006) Supporting midwives to support women. In: L. A. Page and R. McCandlish (eds), *The New Midwifery: Science and Sensitivity in Practice*, 2nd edn (London: Churchill Livingstone/Elsevier).

Deery, R. and Kirkham, M. (2007) Drained and dumped on: the generation and accumulation of emotional toxic waste in community midwifery. In: Mavis Kirkham (ed.), *Exploring the Dirty Side of Women's Health* (London and New York: Routledge), pp.72–83.

Douglas, M. (1966) *Purity and Danger: An Analysis of the Concepts of Pollution and Taboo* (London: Routledge & Kegan Paul).

Dykes, F. (2006) *Breastfeeding in Hospital: Mothers, Midwives and the Production Line* (London: Routledge).

Earle, S., Komaromy, C., Foley, P. and Lloyd, C. (2007) Understanding reproductive loss. Part 2: the moment of death, *The Practising Midwife*, 10(7): 27–30.

Edwards, N. P. (2001) Women's experiences of planning home births in Scotland: Birthing autonomy. Unpublished PhD thesis, University of Sheffield, UK.

Edwards, N. P. (2004) Why can't women just say no? And does it really matter? In: M. Kirkham (ed.), *Informed Choice in Maternity Care* (Basingstoke: Palgrave Macmillan).

Edwards, N. P. (2005) *Birthing Autonomy: Women's Experiences of Planning Home Births* (London: Routledge).

Edwards, N. P and Murphy-Lawless, J. (2006) The instability of risk: Women's perspectives on risk and safety in birth. In: A. Symon (ed.), *Risk and Choice in Maternity Care: An International Perspective* (Edinburgh: Churchill Livingston).

Ehrenreich, B. and Hochschild, A. R. (2002) *Global Woman: Nannies, Maids and Sex Workers in the New Economy* (London: Granta Books).

Frith, H. and Kitzinger, C. (1998) Emotion work as a participant resource: A feminist analysis of young women's talk-in-interaction, *Sociology*, 32(2): 299–320.

Gilligan, C. (1985) *In a Different Voice: Psychological Theory and Women's Development* (Cambridge, MA: Harvard University Press).

Green, J. M, Coupland, V. A. and Kitzinger, J. V. (1998) *Great Expectations: A Prospective Study of Women's Expectations and Experience of Childbirth*, 2nd edn (Hale, Cheshire: Books for Midwives).

Greenhall, F. M. (2001) Doctor–nurse communication in the neonatal intensive care unit: An anthropological analysis, *Journal of Neonatal Nursing*, 7(4): 110–14.

Hamer, M. (1999) Listen to the voice: An interview with Carol Gilligan, *Women: A Cultural Review*, 10(2): 173–84.

Harvey, D. (2005) *A Brief History of Neoliberalism* (Oxford: Oxford University Press).

Higgins, M. R. and Werner-Wilson, R. J. (1997) *What is Emotion Work? How Does it Influence Couples and Families?*, http//www.public.iastate.edu/~rwilson/ CAMFT-97.pdf

Hochschild, A. R. (1983) *The Managed Heart: Commercialization of Human Feeling* (Berkeley, CA: University of California Press).

Hochschild A. R. (2003) *The Commercialization of Intimate Life: Notes from Home and Work* (Berkeley, CA: University of California Press).

Hunter, B. (2000) The emotional work of being a midwife, *Practising Midwife*, 3(2): 34–6

Hunter, B. (2001) Emotion work in midwifery: a review of current knowledge, *Journal of Advanced Nursing*, 34(4): 436–44.

Hunter, B. (2004) Conflicting ideologies as a source of emotion work in midwifery, *Midwifery*, 20(3): 261–72.

Hunter, B. (2006) The importance of reciprocity in relationships between community-based midwives and mothers, *Midwifery*, 22(4): 308–22.

Hunter, B. and Deery, R. (2005) Building our knowledge about emotion work in midwifery and combining and comparing findings from two different research studies, *Evidence-Based Midwifery*, 3(1): 10–15.

Hunter, B. and Smith, P. (2007) Emotional labour: just another buzz word? (Guest Editorial), *International Journal of Nursing Studies*, 44: 859–61.

James, N. (1989) Emotional labour, *Sociological Review*, 37: 15–42.

James, N. (1992) Care = organisation + physical labour + emotional labour, *Sociology of Health and Illness*, 14(4): 488–509.

John, V. and Parsons, E. (2006) Shadow work in midwifery: Unseen and unrecognised emotional labour, *British Journal of Midwifery*, 14(5): 266–8.

Kirkham, M. (1999) The culture of midwifery in the NHS in England, *Journal of Advanced Nursing*, 32(2): 732–9.

Kirkham, M., ed. 2000 *The Midwife–Mother Relationship* (Basingstoke: Palgrave Macmillan).

Kirkham, M. (2003) *Birth Centres: A Social Model for Maternity Care* (Hale, Cheshire: Books for Midwives).

Kirkham, M. and Stapleton, H. (2001) *Informed Choice in Maternity Care: An Evaluation of Evidence Based Leaflets* (York: NHS Centre for Reviews and Dissemination).

Kirkham, M. and Stapleton, H. (2004) The culture of maternity services in Wales and England as a barrier to informed choice. In: M. Kirkham (ed.), *Informed Choice in Maternity Care* (Basingstoke: Palgrave Macmillan).

Kitzinger, S. (1992) Birth and violence against women: Generating hypotheses from women's accounts of unhappiness after childbirth. In: H. Roberts (ed.), *Women's Health Matters* (London: Routledge).

Kitzinger, S. (2006) *Birth Crisis* (Abingdon: Routledge).

Leatherbarrow, B., Winter, P., Macleod, L., Nicoll, A., McNicol, K. and Hoggins, K. (2004) From vision to reality: the development of a community maternity unit, *Midwives*, 7(5): 212–14.

Levy, V. (1999) Midwives, informed choice and power: part 1, *British Journal of Midwifery*, 7(9): 583–6.

Machin, D. and Scamell, M. (1997) The experience of labour using ethnography to explore the irresistible nature of the bio-medical metaphor during labour, *Midwifery*, 13: 78–84.

McClure, R. and Murphy, C. (2007) Contesting the dominance of emotional labour in professional nursing, *Journal of Health Organization and Management*, 21(2): 101–20.

McCourt, C., Stevens, T., Sandall, J. and Brodie, P. (2006) Working with women: developing continuity of care in practice. In: L. A. Page and R. McCandlish, *The New Midwifery: Science and Sensitivity in Practice*, 2nd edn (London: Churchill Livingstone/Elsevier).

McCreight, B. S. (2005) Grief and emotional labour: a study of nurses' experiences in gynae wards, *International Journal of Nursing Studies*, 42(4): 439–48.

McQueen, A. C. H. (2004) Emotional intelligence in nursing work, *Journal of Advanced Nursing*, 47(1): 101–8.

Miller, T. (1998) Shifting layers of professional, lay and personal narratives: Longitudinal childbirth research. In: J. Ribbens and R. Edwards (eds), *Feminist Dilemmas in Qualitative Research* (London: Sage Publications).

Murphy-Lawless, J. (1991) Piggy in the middle: The midwife's role in achieving woman-controlled childbirth, *Irish Journal of Psychology*, 12(2): 198–215.

Murphy-Lawless, J. (1998) *Reading Birth and Death: A History of Obstetric Thinking* (Cork: Cork University Press).

Murphy-Lawless, J. (2006) Birth and mothering in today's social order: the challenge of new knowledges, *MIDIRS Midwifery Digest*, 16(4): 439–44.

Pollock, A. M. (2006) *NHS plc: The Privatisation of Our Health Care* (London and New York: Verso).

Porter, M., and MacIntyre, S. (1984) What is must be best: a research note on conservative or deferential responses to antenatal care provision, *Social Science of Medicine*, 9(11): 1197–1200.

Quipp-Stenson, S. (2007) Disappointed?, *AIMS Journal*, 19(1): 15.

Robinson, J. (2004) Memories are made of this: the midwife effect, *British Journal of Midwifery*, 12(8): 515.

Sandall, J. (1997) Midwives' burnout and continuity of care, *British Journal of Midwifery*, 5(2): 106–11.

Sandall, J., Davies, J. and Warwick, C. (2001) *Evaluation of the Albany Midwifery Practice* (London: Kings College Hospital).

Smith, P. (1988) The emotional labour of nursing, *Nursing Times*, 84(44): 50–1.

Smith, P. (1991) The nursing process: Raising the profile of emotional care in nurse training, *Journal of Advanced Nursing*, 16(1): 74–81.

Smythe, E. (1998) 'Being safe' in childbirth: A hermeneutic interpretation of the narratives of women and practitioners. Unpublished PhD thesis, Massey University, New Zealand.

Staden, H. (1998) Alertness to the needs of others: a study of the emotional labour of caring, *Journal of Advanced Nursing*, 27(1): 147–56.

Stevens, T. (2003) Midwife to mid wif: A study of caseload midwifery. Unpublished PhD thesis, Thames Valley University, London.

Strange, F. (2002) An age of uncertainty: the emotional labour of becoming the parent of a premature baby, *Journal of Neonatal Nursing*, 8(4): 112–17.

van Teijlingen, E. R., Hundley, V., Rennie, A. M., Graham, W. and Fitzmaurice, A. (2003) Maternity satisfaction studies and their limitations: 'What is, must still be best', *Birth*, 30(2): 75–82.

Tones, K. and Green, J. (2002) The empowerment imperative in health promotion. In: J. Dooher and R. Byrt (eds), *Empowerment and Participation: Power, Influence and Control in Contemporary Health Care*, Volume 1 (Dinton, Wiltshire: Quay Books).

Waldenstrom, U. (2004) Why do some women change their opinions about childbirth over time, *Birth*, 31(2): 102–7.

Waldenstrom, U., Hildingsson, I. and Christie, R. I. (2004) A negative birth experience: Prevalence and risk factors in a national sample, *Birth*, 31(1): 17–27.

Walsh, D. (2007) *Improving Maternity Services: Small is Beautiful – Lessons from a Birth Centre* (Oxford: Radcliffe Publishing).

3

Epidurals not Emotions: the Care Deficit in US Maternity Care

Debora Bone

Introduction

In the United States, 99 per cent of all babies are born in hospitals where medical doctors, usually obstetricians, oversee about 92 per cent of the births (Martin et al. 2006). Midwives attend about 8 per cent of US births, including a small number of home births. Within this context of hierarchy and medical authority, maternity nurses provide much of the professional care deemed necessary for a safe, efficient birth, and are the most common attendants of women in labour.[1] Since about 99 per cent of maternity nurses are women, I will use the feminine pronouns 'she' and 'her'.

Traditionally, the maternity nurse's role during the highly charged experience of childbirth includes numerous instances of what Arlie Russell Hochschild (1983) calls 'emotional labour' (for further research on the emotional labour of nurses and midwives, see also: Smith 1992; Hunter 2001, Hunter and Deery 2005; Hunter and Smith 2007). However, contemporary hospital practices have introduced technologies and interventions that have displaced the emotional labour of supporting a woman during natural birth. Widespread use of epidural analgesia and Caesarean section has shifted the focus of the maternity nurse. This article explores how epidurals and other interventions are changing the quality of emotional labour provided in the context of hospital birth in the USA.

Nurses have long performed what I call 'therapeutic emotional labour' (Bone 1997) while carefully managing the layers of emotion called forth during childbirth. However, cumulative structural and treatment-protocol changes within the health care system in the United

States have led to disturbing changes in the meanings and practices of emotional labour. This study suggests that maternity nurses are constrained in providing valuable forms of emotional labour, while tightly managing their own emotions in new contexts of care, resulting in diminished quality of care for women and families during childbirth.

Both the cost containment strategies of market-driven health care, which dominates the US system, and the techno-medical protocols of obstetrical medicine have altered the conditions and values placed on the emotional labour of maternity nurses. Under-recognised yet vital aspects of tending to women during childbirth are being lost or transformed as the organisation of work disallows their practice. Corporate managers prioritise those types of work, skills and knowledges that favour cost containment, medical control and profit making, while eclipsing those types of work that prioritise interpersonal and psychosocial care. Maternity nurses find themselves altering the care they give and clients must often learn how to do without.

During childbirth, a woman becomes extremely vulnerable as hormones and muscles work to open her uterus and allow the newborn to emerge. With effective guidance and support, her emotions can move from fear to courage. The skilled care of an expert labour attendant can help this ancient process to unfold smoothly, allowing her to experience the power and mystery of her own body. Contemporary hospital practices have made it difficult for maternity nurses to provide this kind of care.

The squeeze on nurses as paid providers of care echoes what Arlie Russell Hochschild (2003) has called the contemporary 'care deficit'. She argues that in industrialised countries dominated by the profit-making priorities of capitalism, many health and human services have become commodities, reducing the availability of caregivers and care in both paid and unpaid sectors. Few incentives or resource allocation priorities have been made to ensure adequate interpersonal care in public or private life. She goes on to identify four cultural solutions to the care deficit, of which the 'post-modern solution' is for people to learn to live without much care.

In the medicalised hospital environment, the use of epidural analgesia during labour and delivery could be seen as a powerful, highly embodied metaphor for the post-modern solution to the care deficit. The epidural provides pain relief to the labouring woman and redirects the efforts of the maternity nurse toward technical interventions. Therapeutic emotional labour is displaced by a pharmaceutical solution to the need for support.

Although some would argue that the epidural is an improvement, others challenge that there are significant side effects, as well as important psychosocial losses (Lieberman 1999; Durham 2002). How have the directives for clinical efficiency and cost-effectiveness affected the kind of emotional labour performed by these maternity nurses? What interpersonal skills and nursing expertise are changed when the conditions for their production is altered?

As Hochschild (2003) suggests, the post-modern solution to a structural deficit of care is to deny the need for care and change the way we conceptualise need and well-being. In the context of maternity care, this affects how the emotions surrounding experiences of pain, mothering and birth can be felt and expressed. Nursing care for childbearing women is one example of larger cultural struggles over interpretations of human needs, gendered divisions of labour, and the distribution of social and economic resources.

Therapeutic emotional labour, authoritative knowledge and obstetrical dominance

As part of a larger study of emotion work and nursing (Bone 1997), I interviewed six nurses who provide pre- and perinatal maternity care to women in northern California. The qualitative study included 18 nurses who were either self-identified or identified by others as having well-developed 'emotion skills' and as proponents of providing 'emotional support' to patients. The goal was to learn from the 'experts' what they did, how they spoke about it, and how it fitted in with the overall demands of their work. Both the emotion work[2] of 'doing' interpersonal relations and how they managed their own feelings about their working conditions were explored.

Maternity nurses are often caught between conflicting demands of medical science and technologies, and the commitment to meeting immediate needs of the patients they serve, including interpersonal and emotional dynamics. Benner et al. (2004) has shown that 'knowing the patient' is different from the formalised, data-based knowledge of medical assessment, yet central to clinical judgement. Distinct from the rationalism of statistical analysis, expert nurses acquire skills through bedside practice, gaining knowledge that is specific, embodied and experiential. The resulting skilled 'know-how' and relational expertise (see also Chapter 11) is often less visible or valued by the dominant medical model, yet highly relevant and appreciated by the recipients of care.

When I asked nurses to describe how they provided emotional support, they identified 'ways of being, doing and knowing' that could be considered therapeutic emotional labour. Activities of emotional sensitivity and support are hard to validate and resist standardisation. The nurses themselves tended to take many of them for granted and acknowledged that it was sometimes difficult to distinguish between 'providing emotional support' and 'just chatting'.

For example, gestures of welcoming patients (as highlighted in the preface to this book), making them comfortable, establishing trust, and offering reassurance were seen as commonplace, barely worth mentioning. When I asked nurses to define emotional support, they often prefaced their remarks with 'just', as in 'I just do this or that'. In the hierarchy of tasks and activities, this emotional labour was taken for granted and incidental. It was seen as important for the patients, but outside of the measurement, documentation or accountability of the main work expected by the hospital protocols.

One maternity nurse minimises her skill, while also recognising the value of presence and the non-verbal side of offering reassurance, saying: 'sometimes just being there and listening, sometimes not even speaking but just your physical presence with someone [makes a difference]'. Another maternity nurse emphasises what Davis-Floyd and Davis (1997: 317) call intuition, or immediate cognition. 'I've learned how to have a certain way of behaving, noticing what works, what makes people relax. I can just perceive it in their being when they feel OK.' Describing how she knows the patient, another nurse says: 'It's not a concrete thing always that you can describe. Sometimes it's like a sixth sense, or a perceptiveness. You can get a "take" on somebody and you can't really pinpoint it.'

Knowing how to manage the emotions of a frightened patient or calm the anxiety of a worried woman are skills that maternity nurses learn by doing. This kind of knowledge is passed on informally and becomes part of the 'hands on' repertoire of the expert nurse. An experienced nurse describes this mastery: 'Even as I am doing certain things, there's a manner in which those interventions can be done that can either arouse fear or calmness, or at least neutrality'. The maternity nurse knows how valuable it is to keep her patient calm, even in an emergency:

I calmly just do what needs to be done, and I explain why we're doing it, and get anything I need, give oxygen. There's a way in which I don't get panicked and then usually they don't get panicked, which I think is important, because I think the adrenaline is bad for the baby.

The skills of therapeutic emotional labour are understated, contingent and discretionary. There is a wide range of variation among nurses, settings and situations, yet this work of managing emotions to support the birthing mother reflects 'ways of being, doing and knowing' that are intuitive, relational, experiential and situated. The nurse brings her *self* into the process and learns how best to support the labouring mother.

Not surprisingly, the emotional and interpersonal dimensions of nursing are easily identified with so-called 'innate feminine qualities'. Catherine Lutz (1990: 69) has suggested that the organising category of emotion is so closely associated with the female that 'any discourse on emotion is also, at least implicitly, a discourse on gender'. Binary oppositions of emotion/reason and subjective/objective are embedded in Western assumptions about what counts as knowledge and truth. Emotion and the feminine both have ambivalent status. Both are devalued in relation to reason and thought, and both are exalted as the warm, sensitive and authentic side of human nature, summoned to counteract the cold hard-heartedness of pure science or economics.

In nursing, this ambivalence invokes a classic double bind. On the one hand, women are defined as inherently emotional, and it is seen as their natural proclivity to do emotional labour. On the other hand, emotion is defined as less valuable than reason, so any affirmation of the importance of emotional labour is also an implicit acceptance of inferiority. This paradox is felt throughout the 'care sector' and affects the very ability of occupations like nursing to claim the full status of professional, with its implicit masculine and rational values. Emotional labour and caring are taken for granted, but not seen as 'real work'.

Jordan (1997) and Davis-Floyd and Davis (1997) and others have written extensively about the historical and social construction of authoritative knowledge in childbirth. Ritual practices in the high-tech settings of American birth reinforce medical dominance and serve to exclude the labouring woman's knowledge of her own body and emotions as legitimate. By contrast, advocates of midwifery (Kitzinger 1997; Davis-Floyd and Davis1997) suggest that touch and intuition can be valid sources of authoritative knowledge. Maternity nurses are often caught between their allegiance to techno-medicine and their desire to comprehend and advocate for the patient using the 'soft skills' of emotional labour, intuition, experiential knowledge and caring.

Although women as patients value these often-invisible activities, Jo Murphy-Lawless (1998) examines how contemporary obstetrical practices invoke the threat of death to frighten pregnant women into compliance with the dominant medical paradigm. She shows how women's agency in the birthing process is diminished by a shift of focus to the 'what if' of assessing fetal risk. Construction of the fetus as a separate being reduces the woman to an invisible, inaudible vessel, serving to further medicalise pregnancy. The value, warmth and authority of the connection between mother and infant is pushed aside, replaced by ultrasound images and a focus on the perfect 'designer baby' as the desirable end-product of childbirth. This fetus-centred perspective diminishes the rapport between the labouring woman and her care-givers while giving rationale to bypass the mother's process and interests in order to 'protect the baby'.

The interests of obstetrical medicine to control women during childbirth are reinforced by, and consistent with, the demands of market-driven health care in the United States. Third-party payers (insurance companies) drive policy by determining what gets reimbursed and what doesn't. Health care practices that require extensive diagnostic tests and procedures to avoid malpractice suits, or liberally performing Caesarean sections to avoid 'risks', are common ways to make a profit while keeping labouring women subservient. Resources are rarely allocated that provide adequate recognition and training in the skills of therapeutic emotional labour and other 'soft skills' such as touch, intuition, interpersonal communication, and intimate caregiving.

Maternity nurses respond to the primacy of technology and pharmacology

Contemporary practices that control women during pregnancy and birth must be examined in the context of over two centuries of tension between women and those professing to assist them. Barbara Katz Rothman (1989) is one of many feminist writers to analyse ideology and technology in patriarchal society. She argues that since the Industrial Revolution, mechanical ideals have been applied to motherhood. When labour deviates from the expected trajectory, the mother is deemed inadequate or defective, requiring technological assistance to improve her function. The mechanical extensions of ultrasound, fetal monitoring, intravenous medication and epidural analgesia are seen as ways to improve on the implicit deficiencies of the woman's body.

Building on the work of Davis-Floyd, Jordan and others, Jane Szurek (1997) writes about birth activists in Italy who are challenging medical dominance by affirming alternative, holistic definitions of women in birth and by developing a competing set of authoritative knowledge.

Like the small number of American home births, these and other sites of resistance to medical dominance are made possible by supportive midwifery practices that demonstrate the effectiveness of low-tech, no-drug approaches to childbirth. While many nurses do not have the opportunity to participate in this kind of delivery, all have seen women come in and deliver with very little intervention, and many question the dominant protocols of modern obstetrics.

The majority of American maternity nurses work in hospitals where techno-pharmaceutical practices have increasingly displaced other kinds of labour support. It is not my intention to evaluate the risks and bene-fits of common perinatal technologies and medications. My purpose here is to trace the shift in skills and knowledges expected and used by these nurses, and report their concerns about how the context for and ability to provide certain kinds of emotional labour are being displaced.

In the context of contemporary hospital birth, the maternity nurse is pulled by conflicting demands that tug on her identity and question her allegiances. Depending on the situation, the nurse is alternately expected to serve as assistant to the doctor, protector of the fetus, and advocate for the woman in labour. The maternity nurses interviewed for this study were selected for their commitment and skills in therapeutic emotional labour. The following responses are indicative of the conflict-ing perspectives held by some nurses when facing these multiple demands.

These maternity nurses saw technology and obstetrical medications as ways to speed up the birth process and make it more efficient, but also as an intensification of their work that did not always improve the outcome. For example, one maternity nurse spoke of her ambivalence about the vacuum extractor, a tool that obstetricians attach to the head of a fetus while the mother is pushing out her baby. This instrument is not without risk for both mother and baby, but it can hasten the deliv-ery, thus saving time in a culture where 'time is money'.

> [T]hey used to do a lot of vacuum extractions to help, basically shorten second stage [of labour]. I'd get real frustrated about that. Because I'd get, you know, 'hey this lady is a primip[ara] [ie. a first-time mother], she just needs to push more.' What's the point in pulling the baby out and stressing the baby and making the woman have a big cut on her bottom?

Another maternity nurse described her distaste for central fetal monitor-ing, a technical capability that allows a nurse at a central station to watch the electronic tracings of several fetal hearts at once. In this way, one nurse can oversee several women in labour, spending less time engaged with each mother:

> The new charge nurse was talking about central monitoring and she is planning a proposal for central monitoring. And I said that I worked with [it] in Miami, and I hated it. She looked quite shocked and she said 'Oh, I just love it.' And I said, 'Well, as far as I'm concerned, it just puts you *farther away from the patient.*'   (emphasis added)

Central monitoring allows the maternity nurse's work to be reorganised for efficiency and cost-effectiveness. Some nurses prefer spending less time in the intensity of providing labour support, but other nurses regret the loss of contact.

When asked how increased technologies have changed her work, one respondent noted changes in

> the work itself, there is more to monitor. You may have a machine that is doing it, but you still have to look at the machine and react to what's going on. . . . [W]hat you are doing as a nurse today is far more involved than what you were doing as a nurse twenty years ago because of the technology, because of all that has been learned. . . . [Y]ou've got it right in your face, and if you don't respond to something, you have to be even more on your toes, there's so much more information coming at you. In that respect, I think it is harder. It's less forgiving if you screw up.

The nurse is expected to respond both to the client and to the information communicated by various monitors. Her gestures and comportment incorporate the exigencies of the machine as well as the client. In a sense, the nurse retains and enacts the emotional parts of the nurse/machine complex that are now conjoined in the caregiving project. But in this cyborg moment, the emotions are rarely given primacy.

Donna Haraway (1991) evokes the cyborg as a hybrid of organism and machine to destabilise categories. She calls for a politics that refuses the kind of binary oppositions that have kept woman and emotion the subjugated 'other' to man and reason. Building on a different notion of post-modern from Hochschild, Haraway shows how meanings and priorities are made in specific social/political contexts that are not innocent. Her work examines how the practices of science affect what counts as knowledge. For the nurse and the woman in labour, a cyborg politics might result in hybrid reconfigurations of technological reasoning and emotional insight that better respond to the heterogeneous, contingent and complex realities of birth.

One maternity nurse described the intricacy of making contact with a new client while accomplishing routine clinical tasks:

> There's always the delicate balance between getting those 'initial things' done right away, and letting her know she can labour how she wants to. 'Put on this gown, pee in the cup, get on the monitor, let me get your blood pressure and temperature,' and somehow meeting someone with all those technical things and not make them feel like some *kind of machine.*   (emphasis added)

The nurse sets a tone of openness to the woman's own labour process, while attending to the measurements and machinery of obstetrical care. Beyond either/or, how do nurses adapt and perform emotional labour within the primacy of technology?

Pain management and emotional labour

Pain management during childbirth is one of the greatest challenges for nursing care and for the obstetrical team. There have been techniques for assisting women in labour in every society and historical time period. This support work unfolds according to the display and feeling rules of each culture. Women learn what can or should be felt and expressed, and measures are taken to ensure that they manage the experience in culturally acceptable ways. For centuries, this work was provided primarily by midwives who learned by experience how to strengthen women and lessen sensations of pain.

In the nineteenth century, medical doctors began to use chloroform and ether to provide pain relief during childbirth. Today, epidural analgesia is the predominant form of pain relief. This technology allows medications to be introduced into the tissues surrounding the spinal cord to cause a loss of sensation in the uterine and pelvic regions of the labouring woman. Despite a variety of complications, epidurals are extremely popular and are used by 50 to 90 per cent of women delivering in American hospitals (Vincent and Chestnut 1988; Lieberman 1999; Cartwright and Thomas 2001; Stark 2003).[3]

The use of epidural analgesia to manage pain in labouring women could also be considered as a type of emotion management. In addition to dulling sensations, the epidural can suppress deep feelings that are often part of the labour process. It helps women cope with the discomforts of giving birth and diminishes the need for nursing knowledge and teaching about positions and activities that support the natural birthing process. For example, a client standing up in labour needs someone there to encourage her whereas the epidural requires the patient to lie in bed with the fetal monitor in place. The maternity nurse provides physical and emotional support in either instance, but the two approaches require a different set of skills and actions from the nurse.

Offering her perspective on helping women in labour, one nurse reported that:

> Sometimes they come around when they're ready to deliver. Sometimes they scream the whole time. I don't know. I think ninety-eight percent of the people deliver fine . . . and there's that two percent that are off the curve, you know. And maybe people that are off the curve get the epidural [analgesia] just to shut them up. I think epidurals should be used for hard core physiological [pain] . . . but I think maybe there are those people that get epidurals just because they cannot tolerate any of the pain. I don't know; should we keep track of the emotional support we give people? How would you track it?

'The curve' is a mutable standard that reflects 'normal' expectations for the handling of pain. If nurses and doctors have less time or inclination to assist in other ways, epidural analgesia can be given to supersede other costly forms of emotional support. It is not that the epidural is inexpensive; both forms of care require the attentions of a skilled nurse. The difference is that there is no category for the reimbursement of emotional support. Insurance payers are unwilling to treat emotional labour as an itemised cost. Interestingly, studies have indicated (Atherton et al. 2004) that the strongest determinant of epidural use was insurance type and availability. If the anaesthesiologist could expect reimbursement, the woman was more likely to be given an epidural.

Epidural analgesia alters body, pain and emotion in the interest of efficiency and control. In capitalist societies, dependency and need have become shameful signs of weakness. Many women gladly forgo both the empowerment and the discomforts of natural birth in favour of a culturally acceptable numbing of feeling, reducing as well the need for intensive interpersonal support. In this post-modern context, one maternity nurse expressed disappointment and was resentful to see that her skill was no longer needed:

> I feel like epidurals are like my nemesis. . . . It's just like, 'Don't take my work away from me.' . . . I feel that largely when a woman has an epidural, then really my job is done. Then I become a technician and a recorder of blood pressures and fetal heart rates. There is really not much for me to do at that point. The hospital seems to me to want to streamline everything and categorize and make everything fit into a book. Labour is just the exact opposite of that.

This maternity nurse does not want to reconfigure her skills to those of technician and manager. She is angry that the protocols of techno-medicine are reducing her role; she has no interest in standardising her work.

Post-modern solutions to the care deficit

Over the past 25 years, maternity nurses have experienced increased risk management strategies, cost containment measures, and organisational restructurings that have shifted priorities and altered nurse–patient interactions. The nurses I interviewed expressed frustration and anger about intensifications of work and resultant changes in standards of patient care. With so many tasks, they explained that providing deep emotional support was an ever-lower priority. The nurse's discretionary time to provide personalised care has become a most scarce resource. As one nurse said, 'On busy days you just don't have time to do anything but the technical things that you have to do.' In another context, Karen Davies (1994) has pointed out that the 'clock time' used to organise efficient routines is different from the 'process time' needed for emotional labour (see also Fiona Dykes, Chapter 5). Time spent doing 'invisible work' does not count in production models that treat time as a commodity. Yet, in the words of one respondent,

> There's no substitute for taking time. Time is the key. You can learn how to do a technique fast, . . . but no matter how you have it down with meeting the emotional needs of a patient, it's paced by the patient.

Another respondent spoke of needing to curtail patient demands to match her diminished availability:

[I feel] a kind of impatience, like 'Don't ask for too many things,' I keep saying 'Do you need anything else,' and I try to give it to them, but I have to get across this unconscious message, 'Don't ask for anything else.' You do go away feeling guilty. . . . I've gone home and just sat and cried. A lot of nurses have done that. You know you are not meeting their needs.

The move to bring husband and family support into childbirth settings has provided valuable personal care to birthing women, and also unpaid labour for many of the 'little things' that offer comfort and encouragement. One maternity nurse explained her efforts to teach the family how to provide support:

I ask, 'is there anyone who can come and be with you?' . . . [Then] by me doing with the woman what I do when I'm there, they'll model me; that's basically how I teach them.

On a busy day, these minimally trained helpers provide much of the emotional support that these new mothers get, yet this also represents an added burden for friends and relatives who may lack the necessary experience and skills. If the nurse no longer provides certain kinds of care, the client adapts or learns to do without.

Setting limits and maintaining self-control

It is elusive to measure changes in something as fluid and invisible as emotional labour. Despite changes in treatment protocols and in the organisation of work, neither nurses nor emotions disappear. Nurses tend to be very pragmatic and have adapted to this emotional deskilling, often by shifting from the work of connection to efforts of suppression and distance. For the nurse, personal involvement and caring can be both sources of deep satisfaction and the cause of discomfort and pain. The nurse manages her own emotions, sets boundaries, and negotiates how much to let in and when to close off. In fact, to do this well has long been an invisible skill in nursing.

The nurses interviewed expressed high levels of self-monitoring and self-sanctioning as they spoke of avoiding 'too much attachment'. One nurse used the metaphor of getting 'sucked in' as if the patient's need was a dangerous black hole:

I try to separate myself and tell myself that it's their life. They are making their own choices. It's not my life. . . . I try to [keep distant] because for self-preservation purposes. It's not healthy for me to get *sucked in* above and beyond. I have to really create boundaries so that I can survive and do my job, otherwise I get too entangled, too emotionally entangled. (emphasis added)

A maternity nurse spoke of being reprimanded by a physician for aligning too closely with her patient: 'he thinks I'm a terrible nurse, that I over-identify with my patients, and he doesn't want me to take care of any of his patients' (see also Ruth Deery, Chapter 4). This nurse struggles to keep her *self* separate from the patient; instead she is asked to identify with the detachment of the physician.

For the nurses interviewed, the emotional aspects of caregiving work were highly valued. One nurse said, 'the job wouldn't be very satisfying . . . if you could never feel like you are giving your patients any [emotional] support'. She spoke of the work intensification of recent years, saying:

I went through a stressful time, because I had to make an adjustment personally that I could not expect to do the same things that I did in the past. And I had to let go of doing nursing the way I did. I had to become more technical than I ever had been, and I had . . . to do things faster. That bothered me a lot. I know that I went through a real depression almost, and then finally I had to let go of it. I couldn't do things as thoroughly as I liked. I changed my standards and my expectation. That was very difficult.

This nurse has lowered her expectations about quality care to match the circumstances of her work.

With increased work demands, more technology, but less time, nurses find that providing emotional support is marginalised at best. Nurses varied in what they considered to be acceptable behaviours and expectations. When asked if there was a certain amount of emotional support that she considered routine, one nurse responded:

I think that there's an implied expectation, but I don't think that there's anything that would be considered necessary for the job. I mean, we do have some nurses that come in and they're *just all business*. Just, do this, do that, next patient; nurses who provide, from my point of view little or no emotional support. And that's OK, I mean, there's enough there. It's not that they don't care, it's just that some people are so fixed on what they need to do workwise. They don't feel like that's a necessary component, or at least they don't exhibit that. (emphasis added)

In her study of flight attendants, Hochschild (1983: 129) described the refusal to perform emotional labour as 'going into robot'. For nurses who value therapeutic emotion work, it is painful to watch colleagues choose the post-modern solution of reducing connection. The nurses interviewed are wary of working conditions that prioritise technical procedures and don't allow enough time for meaningful emotional engagement.

Conclusions

Although this was a small sample, these nurses with expertise in providing therapeutic support to women during childbirth, articulated concerns about changes of what is expected and possible. Both the increased techno-medical protocols of contemporary obstetrical care and the organisational efficiencies of managed health care systems have altered the focus of the maternity nurse.

The prevalence of epidural analgesia typifies the post-modern solution to the contemporary care deficit. This pharmaceutical reduction of pain changes the kind of care needed by the woman and alters the expertise provided by the maternity nurse. It shifts both mother and nurse away from the deeper emotional connections forged by the experience of natural childbirth, in favour of the management and control of techno-medical intervention.

For some nurses, it was very disconcerting to no longer be the kind of nurse they wanted to be. Others adapted by setting limits, maintaining protective boundaries, and focusing on 'just doing a job'. In her economic analysis of challenges facing the 'care sector', Nancy Folbre (2006: 17) reflects ominously: 'If you think global warming might cause serious problems, consider the possible consequences of social chilling.' Childbirth is just one moment in the larger context of social arrangements, yet it has great impact on child development and family formation. What new techno-emotionalities might emerge as labour conditions surrounding childbirth continue to evolve? How might the emotional tone set during childbirth affect the next generation of humans coming into life?

Reflective questions

1   Have contemporary working conditions made it problematic for maternity nurses or midwives to feel too deeply? What influences might make it problematic for women to feel too deeply during childbirth?

2   In your own clinical practice, what effects do you see epidurals having on the emotions of the woman and the maternity nurse or midwife?

3   What kinds of knowledge and skills does the expert nurse or midwife use to perform therapeutic emotional labour and how would a novice nurse or midwife learn them?

Notes

1   In the USA, any registered nurse can learn the specialty of maternity nursing and assist the physician in hospital deliveries. Direct-entry and nurse midwives receive an additional degree and licence that allows them to manage vaginal deliveries with levels of independence that vary state by state.

2   Hochschild (1983: 7) distinguishes between 'emotional labour', the management of feeling to create the proper state of mind in others in a wage situation where there is *exchange value*, and 'emotion work', referring to these similar acts in the private context where they have *use value*. However, I would argue that nurses provide both 'therapeutic emotional labour' as an expected part of the job *and* 'emotion work' when managing their own and the feelings of others when on the job, but not as part of the job expectation. For simplicity, in this chapter I use the term 'emotional labour'.

3   There is no national data collected in the US on the use of epidural analgesia during labour. Estimates of epidural prevalence range from 50 to 90 per cent of all deliveries. It is unclear how the Caesarean deliveries are counted in these estimates, since most C-sections come after a 'trial of labour'. The national C-section rate in 2004 was 29 per cent (Martin et al. 2006).

References

Atherton, M. J., Feeg, V. D. and El-Adham, A. F. (2004) Race, ethnicity and insurance as determinants of epidural use: Analysis of a national sample survey, *Nursing Economics*, 22(1): 6–13.

Benner, P., Tanner, C. A., Chesla, C. and Gordon, D. (2004) The phenomenology of knowing the patient. In: S. Gordon, P. Benner and N. Noddings (eds), *Caregiving, Readings in Knowledge, Practice, Ethics, and Politics* (Philadelphia: University of Pennsylvania Press).

Bone, D. (1997) Feeling squeezed: Dilemmas of emotion work in nursing under managed care. Dissertation, University of California at San Francisco, San Francisco.

Cartwright, E. and Thomas, J. (2001) Constructing risk: Maternity care, law and malpractice. In: R. Devries, C. Benoit, E. R. Van Teijlingen and S. Wrede (eds), *Birth by Design: Pregnancy, Maternity Care, and Midwifery in North America and Europe* (New York: Routledge).

Davies, K. (1994) The tensions between process time and clock time in care-work: The example of day nurseries, *Time and Society*, 3(3): 277–303.

Davis-Floyd, R. and Davis, E. (1997) Intuition as authoritative knowledge in midwifery and home birth. In: R. Davis-Floyd and C. F. Sargent (eds), *Childbirth and Authoritative Knowledge* (Berkeley: University of California Press).

Durham, J. (2002) Epidural anesthesia. Internet site, *Birthsong Childbirth Education*: http://onyx-ii.com/birthsong/page.cfm?epidural.

Folbre, N. (2006) Demanding quality: Worker/consumer coalitions and 'high road' strategies in the care sector, *Politics and Society*, 34(1): 11–31.

Haraway, D. J. (1991) *Simians, Cyborgs, and Women: The Reinvention of Nature* (New York: Routledge).

Hochschild, A. R. (1983) *The Managed Heart* (Berkeley: University of California Press).

Hochschild, A. R. (2003) *The Commercialization of Intimate Life* (Berkeley: University of California Press).

Hunter, B. (2001) Emotion work in midwifery: a review of current knowledge, *Journal of Advanced Nursing*, 34(4): 436–44.

Hunter, B. and Deery, R. (2005) Building our knowledge about emotion work in midwifery: Combining and comparing findings from two different research studies, *Evidence Based Midwifery*, 3(1): 10–15.

Hunter, B. and Smith, P. (2007) Emotional labour: Just another buzz word? *International Journal of Nursing Studies*, 44: 859–61.

Jordan, B. (1997) Authoritative knowledge and its construction. In: R. E. Davis-Floyd and C. F. Sargent (eds), *Childbirth and Authoritative Knowledge* (Berkeley, CA: University of California Press).

Kitzinger, S. (1997) Authoritative touch in childbirth: A cross-cultural approach. In: R. E. Davis-Floyd and C. F. Sargent (eds), *Childbirth and Authoritative Knowledge* (Berkeley, CA: University of California Press).

Lieberman, E. (1999) No free lunch on labor day: The risks and benefits of epidural analgesia during labor, *Journal of Nurse Midwifery*, 44(4): 394–8.

Lutz, C. A. (1990) Engendered emotion: Gender, power, and the rhetoric of emotional control in American discourse. In: C. A. Lutz and L. Abu-Lughod (eds), *Language and the Politics of Emotion* (Cambridge: Cambridge University Press).

Martin, J. A., Hamilton, B. E., Sutton, P. D., Ventura, S. J., Menacker, F. and Kirmeyer, S. (2006) Births: Final data for 2004, *National Vital Statistics Reports*, 55(1): 1–101.

Murphy-Lawless, J. (1998) *Reading Birth and Death: A History of Obstetric Thinking* (Bloomington: Indiana University Press).

Rothman, B. K. (1989) *Recreating Motherhood: Ideology and Technology in a Patriarchal Society* (New York: W. W. Norton).

Smith, P. (1992) *The Emotional Labour of Nursing* (Basingstoke: Palgrave MacMillan).

Stark, M. A. (2003) Exploring women's preferences for labor epidural analgesia, *Journal of Perinatal Education*, 12(2): 16–21.

Szurek, J. (1997) Resistance to technology-enhanced childbirth in Tuscany: The political economy of Italian birth. In: R. E. Davis-Floyd and C. F. Sargent (eds), *Childbirth and Authoritative Knowledge* (Berkeley, CA: University of California Press).

Vincent, R. D. and Chestnut, D. H. (1998) Epidural analgesia during labor, *American Family Physician*, 58(8): 1785–92.

4

Community Midwifery 'Performances' and the Presentation of Self

Ruth Deery

Introduction

When practising as a community midwife I remember sharing with my midwifery colleagues that I sometimes found it necessary to 'switch and swap faces' (Bolton 2005: 78) according to the woman I was supporting at the time and the number of visits or clinics I had to undertake that day. I was usually on call for the maternity services twice per week and would almost always be 'called out' for obstetric emergencies, home births, postnatal complications and infant feeding difficulties. I found myself adapting my approach to midwifery in order to cope with the situation I found myself in. I still do this and feel sure that the necessity to 'switch and swap faces' will resonate with other midwives in similar situations. Only last week when I was undertaking a clinical shift one of the midwives said to me, 'you know, Ruth, we're really good actresses as midwives'. She was telling me about a woman she was supporting who was in labour with an intrauterine death and a postnatal woman who had birthed her first baby. She told me she was finding it exhausting having to be 'all smiles in one room and sombre in another room'. Not only did she have to 'switch and swap faces' but she also had to manage her inner feelings according to the particular situation.

Managing and performing emotions in this way, in order to support childbearing women and colleagues, can leave midwives feeling emotionally drained (see Deery and Kirkham 2007). There are also endless reconfigurations in the National Health Service (NHS) and the maternity services, making workplaces more intense than ever. Some of these changes have been unsettling and challenging for midwives and they have learnt to cope with the emotional impact of a constantly changing organisational culture in different ways. There is now ample evidence to support the effects of stress (Sandall 1998) and lack of support (Kirkham and Stapleton 2000; Deery 2003, 2005; Deery and Kirkham 2006) on midwives but there is less interest in the emotional impact of midwifery work. Rather, the focus seems to be on the emotional impact of childbirth on the woman, the baby and her family. Yet in order to 'develop good relationships with different women, midwives clearly need to experience relationships which nurture their own growth' (Deery and Kirkham 2006: 126). Such relationships require an understanding of the 'hard emotion work to bring feeling and face together' (Bolton 2005: 82) in complex organisations such as the NHS.

In this chapter I will explore how community midwives manage and perform emotion on a day-to-day basis, in a midwifery workforce that has reported low morale (Hughes et al. 2002; Deery 2005) and is rapidly dwindling (Ball et al. 2002). The chapter reports some of the findings from an action research study in the north of England that explored community midwives' support needs. Data analysis drew on key ideas from the work of Irving Goffman (1990) and his analysis of the structures of social encounters from the perspective of the dramatic performance. The study had three phases. Phase one involved in-depth interviews with the midwives; it was during the undertaking and analysis of these interviews that the midwives' emotion self-management, or lack of it, became apparent. Phase two involved focus groups, workshops and the introduction of clinical supervision. Phase three comprised final in-depth interviews in order to evaluate the process of clinical supervision.

The eight NHS community midwives participating in the study practised traditional community midwifery in local clinics and women's homes and provided care for women before and after the birth of their baby. The midwives were traditional in the sense that they were geographically situated and worked with the general practitioners who covered that particular area. Each midwife carried a caseload of women but this did not guarantee continuity of care or carer for the women. As practising midwives they all had varied levels of experience. At the time the study was undertaken they were required by hospital policy to update their skills in helping women to birth their babies by working on the delivery suite/labour ward for one week or more every few months. Their working patterns were more flexible than those of their hospital colleagues although their increasing workloads often meant that any flexibility was impossible.

Midwifery work as 'performance'

Every culture has its own particular type of characters (Czarniawska 1997) and the NHS, with its own complex culture, is no exception. In this chapter, midwifery work is viewed as a drama that unfolds in a 'theatrical frame' (Goffman 1974: 124), with midwives as actors. Czarniawska (1997) has examined the drama of bureaucratic life in Swedish organisations, claiming to have uncovered the hidden workings of organisations. She states that the roles of workers are often defined by the demands of the organisation and that there is: 'an increasing theatricality of politics, in which events are scripted and stage-managed for mass consumption and in which individuals and groups struggle for starring roles (or at least bit parts in the dramas of life). This theatricality is a natural . . . feature of our time' (Czarniawska 1997: 33).

This 'theatricality of politics' supports Goffman's (1974) interest in transformed reality and how it can be possible for workers to act in complex layers of their situation or in multiple realities. Thus, the theatricality of midwifery becomes apparent in this chapter as the different performances of the midwives are identified, described and explored. The midwives set the stage; some of them are leading actors and others are followers during their organisational performances.

Goffman (1974, 1990) has analysed the performance aspects of social encounters using the drama metaphor to draw parallels between the stage and performance aspects of social encounters. Although the sociology underpinning Goffman's work is concerned with the nature of the way people organise face-to-face interactions, rather than emotion work, there are nevertheless comparisons that can be made with the way midwives manage their emotions at work. It is not my intention in this chapter to suggest that midwives switch themselves 'on and off' from one performance to another in a reductionist manner. Rather, I explore how they can 'glide from one performance of face-work to another, sometimes matching feeling and face with situation and at others merely maintaining face' (Bolton 2005: 84).

Midwives as 'emotional labourers'

Midwives who interact with different women on a continuous basis have to contend with different types of emotion work (Hunter 2004), which often involves 'performing' or taking control of their composure or emotions. For example, when midwives engage with women in longer interactions the consequence is longer emotional composure, which requires greater attention to performance and emotional stamina (Hochschild 1983) on the part of the midwife. The midwife I talk about in the introduction to this chapter is alluding to sustained composure and emotional stamina that she thinks makes her a 'good actress'. Longer, more intense interactions also mean that women will often disclose further information about themselves, thus making it harder for the midwife to avoid showing her own personal feelings (Smith 1992), yet drawing them further into the developing relationship. In this situation the midwife has no option but to listen to the woman, managing and adapting her performance, including her own emotional layers, at the same time. Bolton (2005) has produced a useful typology of workplace emotion (p. 93), highlighting that there are several motivations linked to an individual's emotion management performance in an organisation. These motivations are also constantly emerging and changing according to different workplace situations. Therefore, a midwife's 'emotional armour can be donned in a great many ways' (Hochschild 1998: 10).

When the data were analysed using voice-centred relational methodology (Mauthner and Doucet 1998), four different but interrelated aspects of the midwives' roles were identified (see Figure 4.1). Further analysis revealed how they were expected to relate to, and develop partnerships

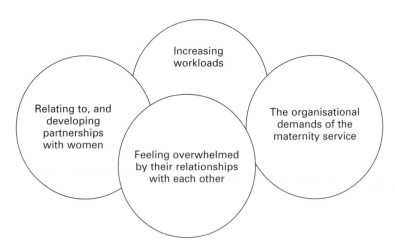

Figure 4.1 Interrelated aspects of community midwives' roles

with clients, when they themselves were inadequately prepared for this aspect of their role. The midwives articulated feeling overburdened by the organisational demands of the maternity service and their increasing workloads. Their words also suggested that they were overwhelmed by their relationships with each other. As a result, the midwives were forced to adapt their behaviour in ways that made their work easier (Lipsky 1980).

I will now consider each of these interrelated aspects in turn, using the midwives' words to illustrate how they adapted their performances according to the organisational situation they were working in.

Relating to, and developing partnerships with women

One of the midwives suggested that when she had to deal with complex issues within the midwife–mother relationship she used a coping strategy that involved her 'putting on a front' in order that she could deal with the situation:

> I had to psych myself up to go into someone particularly if their circumstances were sensitive or there was a language barrier . . .

The ability to 'psych one's self up' (Van Maanen and Kunda 1989: 55) (or down for that matter) could be described as a coping strategy performance. The midwife's words above suggest that she had to calibrate her performance in order to deal with different workplace situations. Another midwife in the work team had learned to cope by ensuring that she always put on a polished performance for her colleagues so that they were not able to detect her stress:

> people think that you cope and think that you are alright . . . this is something you often perpetuate because you wouldn't have them know anything else . . . I think there are times inside when I've thought 'god if my colleagues knew how I was feeling right now' . . . you've got this image haven't you . . . you've got to keep going . . .

This accords with Goffman's (1990) analysis, which sees a person's 'self' as a socialised entity, created in and through social interaction. This midwife resorts to 'impression management' of a deceptive nature so that her self-presentation is perceived by her colleagues as 'coping'. Those who let their masks slip (Fineman 2003), or show signs of any cracks, risk leaking their feelings and this might disrupt the 'united front' (Goffman 1990) put on by the midwives. As Fineman (2003: 37) states, this is how 'professional image and mystique is maintained'.

Another of the midwives reported that having two children of her own during her midwifery career had enhanced her personal and professional development and as a result increased her interpersonal confidence as a midwife:

> I just think having my own children, just being more mature . . . I don't worry about how I'm going to get on with women now and I know I have a good relationship with 99.9% of them . . . there's always a clash with one in a thousand . . . but I think my relationships are good and I've just become a better communicator with experience and a bit of awareness.

This increase in confidence and communication skills meant that she was personally energised by midwifery and was able to judge the level of involvement required in her interactions. One of the midwives, who had been a community midwife for many years, reflected on how midwifery work used to be and how the organisation of midwifery now meant that time spent with women had been reduced to a minimum (see also Debora Bone, Chapter 3). The lack of opportunity to perform friendship with women was seen as a retrograde step by this midwife, who had enjoyed giving that 'personal touch':

> we used to spend hours with them in their homes and, you know, you were really their friend . . . you were their friend in the end . . . but you're so busy now that personal touch is lost.

The midwives stated that there was only so much of a woman's emotional distress that they could listen to and that deciding when this point had been reached posed difficulties for them. One midwife reported undertaking an antenatal interview with a woman who had disclosed that she had had a termination at 22 weeks' gestation, more than ten years ago. The midwife had found this disclosure distressing and stated that 'just her telling me her experience of that was quite traumatic really'. This midwife had clearly been alarmed by this encounter which had required a genuine sincere performance on her part. This midwife also informed me that this was the first time she had told someone about how she had experienced feelings of distress and helplessness following such disclosures. This 'holding in performance' is reminiscent of 'practitioners keeping their emotional lids on tight' (Bond and Holland 1998: 65) to their detriment. The tightness of the lid, and whether its pressure is having a detrimental effect, will depend on the midwife's interpersonal skills, her chosen level of involvement and personal closeness to the woman.

Emotional engagement

One of the midwives reported that the effort she put into continuity of care for the women was more rewarding within team midwifery than traditional community midwifery. More importantly, this midwife appeared to use the challenge of emotion work in midwifery to improve her clinical practice and saw emotional engagement with women as beneficial for midwifery as well as her own personal development. Rather than withdrawing emotionally from situations this midwife preferred to be 'psychologically present' (Kahn 1992) with women. Therefore, rather than giving an empty performance (Bolton 2005: 79) this midwife experienced emotion work as a source of energy:

> I found the continuity for myself was good . . . I found that I knew my women better . . . I got to know the antenatal women, got to know them postnatally . . . so I found it was good for me.

Experiencing emotion work as energising accords with work undertaken by Henderson (2001) who reported the degree of emotional engagement/detachment associated with nurses' work is linked to the degree of satisfaction experienced in the emotional rewards of their work with patients. Bolton's (2000, 2001) analysis also reports nurses experiencing emotion work as satisfying. The midwife's words therefore suggested that the emotional engagement that continuity of care brought to her midwifery work was valued and she seemed to achieve a greater sense of job satisfaction than some of her peers. Another of the midwives reported that it was important to spend time with women and her words suggest that she actively sought and identified women's needs:

> I'll think I'm glad I spent time with her doing that . . . it made a difference to her and I really do feel if you invest . . . particularly early on with these women . . . if you invest some time with them and listen to them they find their feet so much faster . . . if you just spend that time initially . . .

However, this midwife's words also implied the importance she placed on making herself available for women, the organisation of midwifery care and her workload. A different midwife talked about the way in which another midwifery colleague appeared to withdraw emotionally from situations, preferring to perform her midwifery work in a manner that detached her from women. When she observed colleagues becoming 'fully immersed' (Bolton 2005: 80) in the midwife–mother relationship, this was at odds with, and may even have felt threatening to, her preferred way of working:

> I think she has always had a problem with the way that I am with women . . . she thinks that I take too much on . . . she thinks that I am too friendly with them . . . that I should cut off . . . but I don't see my job as just for nine months . . . I see it as a job that goes on forever . . . and with other pregnancies . . . she thinks that you should forget about it at the end of the day and not have anything more to do with it [the job] . . . but maybe women are a bit more . . . I don't like to use the word demanding because I don't think they are . . . maybe their expectations of us are greater . . . and for some of the older midwives they prefer to work more traditionally . . . whereas rather than turning it round on the women and saying 'well what do you want to do about this?' . . . it's been more that she has told them what to do.

The approach to care described above by one of the midwives (and also by the nurses in Debora Bone's chapter) draws attention to midwives' ability to be able to use practical midwifery skills and midwifery knowledge at the same time. The data seem to suggest that the midwife who was described seemed to prefer to ignore any midwifery knowledge that she had acquired and was likely to resort to 'traditional' ways of working as opposed to using her midwifery expertise and knowledge. This approach to care was also likely to leave all problem-solving and decision-making processes to the doctor or other midwives (Deery 2003, 2005). This midwife was unlikely to be intellectually challenged through the midwife–mother relationship, preferring instead a task-orientated performance (Deery 2003, 2005).

Practical and intellectually challenging performances

Some of the midwives experienced interpersonal relationships with women as lasting and of value. One of them reported that 'some people have got it [ability to engage] and some haven't', implying that some midwives are more skilled than others when dealing with women on an interpersonal level.

> I just feel that I can give them . . . I've got quite good at assessing what [the women] need and listening to her about her needs and it's all about communication skills or if I can't listen to her because I can't understand her . . . then assessing her in different ways . . . and then build up the relationship accordingly . . .

This midwife's words are important as they seem to suggest a desire to perform midwifery work on a practical level as well as performing the midwifery role so that she became intellectually challenged and was thus energised by her performance as a midwife. Some of the midwives were able to perform their role within the dynamics of the midwife–mother relationship in a problem-solving way. These midwives appeared to find their performances and relationships with women intellectually challenging and a source of energy, reiterating that emotion work can be performed with satisfaction as well as with negative consequences. Such performances demonstrate midwifery skills that are under-recognised and rarely written about within the profession. The consequence of this is that these skills are not role-modelled and adopted by other midwives and transferred from midwife to midwife.

The organisational demands of the maternity service

One of the midwives provided a good example of the stressful effects of having to respond to the organisational needs of the maternity service whilst suffering the negative consequences of emotion work. In her interview she describes working a 12-hour shift and caring for a woman with an intrauterine death. Her words below suggest physical and emotional exhaustion as well as expressing anxiety around not remembering some of the practicalities of the job:

> I went home and I sat in the chair for about an hour and a half . . . just like zombified . . . thinking about what had gone on . . . and if I had done everything . . .

This midwife's words suggest that her anxiety was more related to whether she had 'done everything', indicating that she was probably more concerned about the needs of the maternity service as an organisation rather than the needs of the woman she was attending. This midwife appeared concerned that she had completed the necessary paperwork and informed the woman of hospital protocol around the death of her baby. A defensive care performance had provoked anxiety within the midwife, taking precedence over engaging emotionally with the woman. This approach then resulted in the midwife feeling drained of all energy (see also Deery and Kirkham 2007).

One of the midwives reported that 'we have to do as we are told', suggesting performances that entailed compliance, hierarchical working relationships and a need to meet organisational demands as a priority. Another midwife reported how her role as a community midwife meant that she often met the demands of the organisation by working on her days off and during the evening:

> we were so badly off for staff . . . I worked my days off . . . two out of three weeks . . . because we were so short-staffed . . .

This same midwife suggested that the relentless pressure of coping with situations that required immediate attention, and that were stressful, affected her performance as a midwife:

> you don't think it's getting to you and then something else gets on top . . . work's a big part of the picture . . .

The performances of community midwives and the demands that these placed on them appear to have limited their ability to perform other roles so that the boundaries of their personal and work life become blurred, making it difficult for them to sustain their acts.

Feeling overwhelmed by their relationships with each other

The demands the organisation placed on the midwives and their increasing workloads left them little space for concentrating on their relationships with each other and on ways in which each of them could build on their contribution to the work team. Previous literature has identified relationships between doctors and midwives as a potential source of conflict (Curtis 1991; Murphy-Lawless 1991). However, there is now evidence (Hughes et al. 2002; Deery 2003; Hunter 2004, 2005) that this is far from reality and that the problem now lies between midwives themselves (Deery 2003; Hunter 2004, 2005).

The strain on working relationships within a work culture that places emphasis on meeting the demands of the organisation can become a source of exhaustion and stress for midwives. A culture that demands efficient 'service and sacrifice' (Kirkham 1999) can take its toll on midwives, with working relationships suffering. Their words suggested that they were unable to 'connect' with each other and that they deferred their own needs, again 'holding in' feelings. This was summed up as:

> midwives are their own worst enemies . . . we don't back each other up . . . it was very stressful . . . very stressful because we were . . . we had two people's work to do in a day basically and with the best will in the world you can only be in one place at once can't you . . . and then the mobile phones . . . meetings to attend . . . .study leave . . . we were getting . . . arguing amongst ourselves . . . niggly . . . bickering . . . one person felt another wasn't doing enough . . . the situation put us under such pressure.

Increasing workloads

Despite the fact that their caseloads had increased enormously, some of the midwives still insisted on performing a work ethic 'above and beyond' what would normally be expected within their job description. One of the midwives, however, chose to don her 'emotional armour' (Hochschild 1998) differently. Her reluctance to become involved with extra commitments suggested that she wanted to protect herself from the stress that she observed in her colleagues. This self-protection added another dimension to the performance of the midwifery role because, as a result, this midwife sometimes experienced feelings of isolation within the team. Her words suggested that the other midwives in the team attempted to intimidate her:

> Well I think they're wrong, I think they want to be up to their arm pits in work you see, they want to do things on the computer at home at night, like working out protocols and things, well I don't . . . and yet because you don't feel that you're involved all the time they make you feel guilty.

In a culture of economic rationing of resources the midwives appeared to prefer projecting an image of 'a good midwife is a busy midwife' (Robinson 1995). However, this style of working, often created through an organisation's attempts to instil a particular set of values (Fineman 2003), means that midwives often resort to sick leave because they are unable to undertake or perform changed working practices. One of the midwives reported an increasing number of midwives taking sick leave because of stress, probably associated with increasing workloads:

> I think it is very worrying . . . I'm extremely worried about the increased number of nervous breakdowns . . . and I'm not talking about minor ones . . . I'm talking mega ones . . . and it's all to do with stress . . .

Changed working practices thus meant that midwives took more sick leave and as a result the midwives left to carry the caseload within the team were forced to cover their colleagues' work in their absence. This then led to more stress and ultimately more members of the team taking sick leave.

Midwives who balance well

Engaging in reciprocal relationships with women, colleagues and the organisation demanded 'tough, emotional hard-labour' (Fineman 2003: 35) that often left midwives having to 'pick the right balance' (Levy 1999) in order to calibrate their performances.

Moreover, the midwives appeared to engage with women at different levels in order to cope with organisational pressures and the emotion work that was demanded. Thus, the ability to glide from one performance to another may operate as a safety valve for midwives, helping them to 'make conscious choices based on their emotional needs and on their understanding of what they can handle at a particular time' (Carmack 1997: 141). Task-based performances became the favoured way of working for most of the midwives because this meant that they could distance themselves from women, making it easier to complete their work within the constraints of the organisation. Such emotional detachment limited and fragmented the development of relationships as they tried to fit women into the bureaucracy of the maternity services. Indeed, they appeared to reach a point at which their increasing workloads precluded women's needs being met and then emotion work became either impossible, could not be entered into, or became a stressor and not a source of energy. The midwives who appeared to balance well in this study were sensitive to their own personal emotional needs, and they chose their level of engagement according to the situation they were presented with at a particular time. They were also able to constantly rebalance their work situation and rather than experiencing emotion work negatively they found their work to be a personally enhancing experience. However, in times of heightened anxiety or stressful situations, midwives can lose the ability to manage and express their feelings effectively to the point where they are no longer able to empathise with women and their colleagues and their work becomes routine, ritualised and depersonalised.

Table 4.1 attempts to set out the parameters of negative and positive

Table 4.1 Midwives' ways of emotional engagement in a bureaucratic context and their subsequent effects

Positive emotional engagement	Negative emotional engagement
• Midwives are able to balance their relationships with women. These are lasting and valued.	• Midwives' relationships with women are fragmented and experienced as 'psychologically draining' and stressful.
• Midwives behave autonomously and are able to think independently.	• In the absence of autonomy midwives become subversive and obedient.
• Midwives value spending time with women and understand continuity of carer. They actively seek and identify women's needs and invite feedback from them.	• Midwifery work becomes task-orientated with decision making left to the doctor. Midwives become swamped by the demands of midwifery and selective with their women.
• Midwives enjoy the complexity of midwifery and thrive on stimulation, challenge and change. They also value emotion work.	• Midwives use their professional power rather than communication skills to set the parameters of the relationship and they become detached from women.
• Midwives are intellectually challenged by their work and are able to use their midwifery knowledge and practical skills together.	• Midwives feel 'wrung out', 'drained', 'empty' and like wet rags (see Deery and Kirkham, 2007) and are unable to use their midwifery knowledge and practical skills together.
• Midwives are able to rebalance their relationships in order to sustain positive emotional engagement.	• Midwives feel a need to be needed and their emotional capacity becomes untenable.
• Midwives experience their work and their colleagues as a source of energy.	• Midwives experience their work and their colleagues as a one-way draining of emotional energy.

emotional engagement as reported by the midwives who participated in this study. In no way are the differentiations meant to be black and white or a tidy typology. Rather they represent opposite ends of the spectrum with the potential for a balancing of both somewhere in the middle.

Conclusion

The data presented in this chapter suggest that midwives combine many different performances into their daily work routines. Although they were in an ideal position as community midwives to offer an individualised approach to women, the midwives were constrained by excessive organisational demands and limited resources. As the midwife in the introduction to this chapter suggested, the pressure to meet organisational demands meant that they had to calibrate and control their performances, which required considerable emotional energy on their part. Calibrating their performances in this manner also meant that working relationships were affected and the midwives reported making choices about whether or not to engage with each other and with women. Thus, they were unable 'to carry out the performances required for an organisationally allocated role whilst holding onto their own sense of identity' (Bolton 2005: 85). This situation resulted in their viewing midwifery negatively and becoming swamped and selective with their increasing workloads. The needs of women were perceived by the midwives as demanding highly polished, well-informed performances which also required tough, 'emotional hard-labour' (Fineman 2003: 35). Rather than viewing relationships with women as a challenge, and experiencing them as energising, the midwives experienced their relationships with women as onerous: a one-way draining of emotional energy where it was impossible to feel enthusiastic about their work.

In an NHS culture that insisted that organisational demands were met, this meant that the midwives had little time to concentrate on their relationships with women and each other. Neither were they able to concentrate on their personal and professional development. Indeed, the midwives spent most of their time at work participating in 'impression management' which resulted in performances that led to a one-way draining of emotional energy rather than a fulfilling, energising process.

Relationships that are starved of positive energy are not reciprocal or fulfilling for midwives, or childbearing women, and often result in a preference for the dominant 'power-over' style of working (Casey 1995; Gallant et al. 2002). The insights provided by the midwives into their working lives suggest that emotion work impinges not only on their relationships with women but also with their peers and their relationships at home. Clearly, a greater understanding of emotion work is essential for midwives and managers within the NHS in the UK if midwives are to 'perform' effectively and better understand their emotional intelligence (Hunter and Smith 2007) whilst retaining their own sense of identity.

Reflective questions

1   How do you *feel* about your midwifery work? Which are your own favoured midwifery 'performances'? Consider different situations at work that could be stressful and personally satisfying for you.

2   Which emotions do you feel the most need to 'manage' and why?

3   Which aspects of your midwifery work do you find difficult and how do you cope with them? Compare your answer with the aspects of midwifery work that are satisfying for you.

References

Ball, L., Curtis, P. and Kirkham, M. (2002) *Why Do Midwives Leave?* (London: The Royal College of Midwives).

Bolton, S. C. (2000) Who cares? Offering emotion work as a 'gift' in the nursing labour process, *Journal of Advanced Nursing*, 32: 580–6.

Bolton, S. C. (2001) Changing faces: nurses as emotional jugglers, *Sociology of Health and Illness*, 23: 85–100.

Bolton, S. C. (2005) *Emotion Management in the Workplace* (Basingstoke: Palgrave Macmillan).

Bond, M. and Holland, S. (1998) *Skills of Clinical Supervision for Nurses: A Practical Guide for Supervisees, Clinical Supervisors and Managers* (Buckingham: Open University Press).

Carmack, B. J. (1997) Balancing engagement and detachment in caregiving, *Image: Journal of Nursing Scholarship*, 29: 149–3.

Casey, A. (1995) Partnership nursing: influences on involvement of informal carers, *Journal of Advanced Nursing*, 22: 1058–62.

Curtis, P. A. (1991) Midwives in hospital: work, emotion and the labour process. Unpublished PhD thesis, University of Manchester.

Czarniawska, B. (1997) *Narrating the Organization, Dramas of Institutional Identity* (London: University of Chicago Press).

Deery, R. (2003) Engaging with clinical supervision in a community midwifery setting: an action research study. Unpublished PhD thesis, University of Sheffield.

Deery, R. (2005) An action research study exploring midwives' support needs and the effect of group clinical supervision, *Midwifery*, 21: 161–76.

Deery, R. and Kirkham, M. (2006) Supporting midwives to support women. In: L. Page and R. McCandlish (eds), *The New Midwifery: Science and Sensitivity in Practice* (London: Elsevier).

Deery, R. and Kirkham, M. (2007) Drained and dumped on: the generation and accumulation of emotional toxic waste in community midwifery. In: M. Kirkham (ed.), *Exploring the Dirty Side of Women's Health* (London: Routledge).

Fineman, S. (2003) *Understanding Emotion at Work* (London: Sage Publications).

Gallant, M. H., Beaulieu, M. C. and Carnevale, F. A. (2002) Partnership: an analysis of the concept within the nurse–client relationship, *Journal of Advanced Nursing*, 40: 149–57.

Goffman, E. (1974) *Frame Analysis: An Essay on the Organization of Experience* (Boston, MA: Northeastern University Press).

Goffman, E. (1990) *The Presentation of Self in Everyday Life* (Harmondsworth: Penguin; first published in 1959).

Henderson, A. (2001) Emotional labor and nursing: an under-appreciated aspect of caring work, *Nursing Inquiry*, 8: 130–8.

Hochschild, A. R. (1983) *The Managed Heart: Commercialization of Human Feeling* (Berkeley, CA: California, University of California Press).

Hochschild, A. R. (1998) Sociology of emotion as a way of seeing. In: G. Bendelow and S. J. Williams (eds), *Emotions in Social Life* (London: Routledge).

Hughes, D., Deery, R. and Lovatt, A. (2002) A critical ethnographic approach to facilitating cultural shift in midwifery, *Midwifery*, 18: 43–52.

Hunter, B. (2004) Conflicting ideologies as a source of emotion work in midwifery, *Midwifery*, 20: 261–72.

Hunter, B. (2005) Emotion work and boundary maintenance in hospital-based midwifery, *Midwifery*, 21: 253–66.

Hunter, B. and Smith, P. (2007) Emotional labour: Just another buzz word? Guest Editorial, *International Journal of Nursing Studies*, 44: 859–61.

Kahn, W. A. (1992) To be fully there: psychological presence at work, *Human Relations*, 45: 321–9.

Kirkham, M. and Stapleton, H. (2000) Midwives' support needs as childbirth changes, *Journal of Advanced Nursing*, 32: 465–72.

Kirkham, M. (1999) The culture of midwifery in the National Health Service in England, *Journal of Advanced Nursing*, 30(3): 732–9.

Levy, V. (1999) Protective steering: a grounded theory study of the processes involved when midwives facilitate informed choice in pregnancy, *Journal of Advanced Nursing*, 29: 104–12.

Lipsky, M. (1980) *Street-Level Bureaucracy: Dilemmas of the Individual in Public Services* (New York: Russell Sage Foundation).

Mauthner, N. and Doucet, A. (1998) Reflections on a voice-centred relational method: analysing maternal and domestic voices. In: J. Ribbens and R. Edwards (eds), *Feminist Dilemmas in Qualitative Research, Public Knowledge and Private Lives* (London: Sage Publications).

Murphy-Lawless, J. (1991) Piggy in the middle: the midwife's role in achieving woman-controlled childbirth, *Irish Journal of Psychology*, 12: 198–215.

Robinson, A. (1995) Transformative 'cultural shifts' in nursing: participatory action research and the 'project of possibility', *Nursing Inquiry*, 2: 65–74.

Sandall, J. (1998) Occupational burnout in midwives: new ways of working and the relationship between organisational factors and psychological health and well being, *Risk Decision and Policy*, 3: 213–32.

Smith, P. (1992) *The Emotional Labour of Nursing* (Basingstoke: Palgrave Macmillan).

Van Maanen, J. and Kunda, G. (1989) 'Real feelings': emotional expression and organizational culture, *Research in Organizational Behaviour*, 11: 43–103.

5

'No time to care': Midwifery Work on Postnatal Wards in England

Fiona Dykes

Introduction

In this chapter I focus upon the temporal tensions and dilemmas experienced by midwives in relation to supporting postnatal women in the hospital setting in England. By temporal, I mean relating to time. I commence by highlighting the ways in which the factory ethos and the centrality of the mechanical clock have influenced hospital culture. I highlight key literature that focuses upon the emotional costs of 'processing the public' for health and social care workers. I draw upon my own critical ethnographic research within postnatal wards in the north of England to highlight the experience of doing midwifery work at the end of the medical production line. I then elaborate upon the experiences for postnatal women of 'being processed' by midwives and, finally, I emphasise the need to restore caring rhythms and relationality between midwives and women.

Development of a clockwork culture

To understand the organisational culture of the hospital it is important to acknowledge the affiliations between the hospital and factories and the place of the mechanical clock in regulating activities in both. Gray (1993) observes that during the Industrial Revolution in Europe, as capitalism, mechanisation and the requirement for controlled production methods grew, the need for precise timing, measurement and consistency was firmly established. The construction of the mechanical clock provided a perfect tool to connect the imperatives of industrial production, measurement, timing and monitoring of factory workers.

Cipolla (1967) argues that it was during the seventeenth century, when the scientific revolution reached a zenith in Western Europe, that scientists saw the clock as 'the machine *par excellence*' (1967: 57). Their growing interest in the clock led to its rapid technological sophistication and people increasingly timed activities that they would never have considered timing before. Clocks were changing ways of thinking as they replaced the variable times, associated with the seasons, with a meticulously measured time that superseded the former.

What evolved during the Industrial Revolution was the notion of mechanical clock or linear time. Kahn (1989) argues that linear time is 'pitched towards the future' and is centred around the notion of production which, in the factory, not only overrides closeness to natural body rhythms and flows, but with shift work even erases day and night distinctions. In contrast, she asserts that cyclical time is a bodily, rhythmic time that is a part of one's ontology and not separate and 'outside' like linear time. It relates to the 'organic cycle of life' in which one is 'living within the cycle of one's own body' (1989: 21).

The deep penetration of the clock in society and the mutual dependence, in the West, between the clock and technological 'progress' is emphasised by Simonds (2002: 569): 'A cultural ethos (capitalist, technocratic, bureaucratic, and psychologically individualistic) makes time keeping relevant, and, the more it develops such foci, the more it creates technology to assess, to measure, to control'.

The super-valuation of time reached into many aspects of the lives of English people and, as Millard (1990) argues, the clock developed an 'unparalleled position as a symbol of science, discipline, and the co-ordination of human effort' (1990: 217). In England, it could be said that the predominant icon is 'Big Ben', an enormous clock and bell situated in the heart of London and a central attraction for visitors from around the world.

The twentieth century brought with it a dramatic increase in hospitalisation of women during childbirth and postnatal recovery, and the hospital, like the factory, was a place in which the principles of linear time and associated routines and schedules became central to efficient production.

Midwifery work at the end of the medical production line

In the UK, postnatal care, for most women, takes place initially in the hospital. The length of stay may vary from a few hours to several days.

Postnatal care has low status in the techno-medical hierarchy, often being described as the 'Cinderella' of the maternity service, reflecting its impoverished status in terms of resources and staffing (Ball 1994; Garcia et al. 1998; Royal College of Midwives 2000; Singh and Newburn 2000).

I conducted a postnatal ward critical ethnographic study, completed in 2004, in two fairly typical consultant-led maternity units in the north of England. The underpinning theoretical perspective that I applied stemmed from critical medical anthropology, a form of anthropology that opposes the medicalisation of everyday life in contemporary society and critiques medicine as an institution. It sees biomedicine as a form of power, domination and social control and challenges reductionist approaches to health care and their underpinning mind–body dualism (Csordas 1988). The study connected a macro, political economy of health perspective with a micro perspective, focusing upon organisational cultures and the lived experiences of individuals within specific cultural milieux.

The research took place on maternity wards that served antenatal and postnatal women. Both hospitals served populations that spanned higher to lower socio-economic occupational groupings. Thirty-nine midwives and 61 postnatal women consented and subsequently participated. The study focus involved observation of interactions between midwives and mothers, related to support with breastfeeding, and follow-up interviews with both groups (Dykes 2005a, 2005b, 2006). This chapter focuses very specifically upon the organisational culture and working conditions for midwives in the postnatal ward setting, and the ways in which these conditions affected encounters between midwives and the women that they were endeavouring to support.

Midwives' experiences

The postnatal wards represented the final stop on the medical production line with midwives working at the end of a fast medical conveyor belt. Midwives powerfully illustrated their dissatisfaction with their workplace culture by their actions and body language as they passed me by. They would often 'sigh' and made comments indicating their relief at completing aspects of their work, surviving the shift and going off duty soon. They frequently commented upon the extreme busyness of the wards and the temporal pressures this created:

> There isn't the time needed to help women, let alone give them appropriate breastfeeding support . . . you can't do that when you're

busy. You might have several antenatals, an early labourer, post sections and we're even the over spill for gynae . . . You just can't do it.   (Virginia)

The rationing of time led to midwives being preoccupied with processing their work as efficiently as possible, as also observed in related ethnographies (Street 1992; Kirkham and Stapleton 2001a; Stapleton et al. 2002; Varcoe et al. 2003; Hunter 2004). The sense of urgency was, in part, based on the constant unpredictability of their daily work situation. They could be called to delivery suite, theatre or antenatal clinic when needed, at a moment's notice, leaving the post-natal ward depleted of staff. This unpredictability removed from the midwives any sense of safety, security or stability. At any time an emergency could arise, particularly with the antenatal women, creating even more unpredictability:

You never know when you might be moved . . . can you really get to know anyone when you may be shifted off at a moment's notice . . . staff can be working on the ward, clinic, delivery and theatre all in one day. On top of that there aren't enough staff and therefore we can only try to give breastfeeding advice but often that's not enough. (June)

Being moved was disruptive not only for the midwife who relocated but for those left on the postnatal ward:

You can start off with only one room and an hour later you could have the whole ward. So you can't just take your time . . .   (Linda)

The ways in which the working patterns hindered forming of rela-tionships were also articulated:

My problem today is that I've come on at 8.15. I have to cover clinic later, so if I came on at 7.15 and then covered clinic to 5 it would be too long a day. So . . . I come on at 8.15. I don't get a report, I know nothing about the women and I'm not even here to hand over to the next shift. What sort of continuity is that? The system needs to be changed.   (Virginia)

Several staff members commented upon the effects of the 'system' upon retention of midwives:

The staff are draining away. It's the system we have here. It's disruptive. There's no flexibility. We are losing experienced staff. There's low morale . . . nobody knows what is going on. They're here, there and everywhere.   (Jade)

There's currently a mass exodus of staff here. They just can't stand it, the way they work here . . . Someone can come on in the morning and move to clinic or delivery, often with a minute's notice. It's making them very insecure and there's no ownership whatsoever. I mean they don't feel a part of this ward at all . . . you are moving round so fast you can't think.   (Jenny)

The midwives thus presented a picture of temporal pressures, lack of control over their working conditions, inability to form meaningful relationships with women, inflexibility and insecurity. Neither midwives nor mothers had any real influence over whom they encountered in hospital. The combination of shortage of time plus unpredictability that contributed to a rushed, chaotic and fragmented approach to care is also described in other related midwifery contexts (Ball 1994; Kirkham 1999; Kirkham and Stapleton 2000; Ball et al. 2002; Hunter 2004).

Being processed: women's experiences

Under the busy conditions described, mothers were inevitably reluctant to ask for help. They noticed and commented on the temporal pressures upon midwives:

The midwives seem to be, you know . . . um . . . spread very thinly and they don't have much time.   (Alison)

They seem to be pressured, panicky and anxious.   (Bryony)

They do seem to be so busy and understaffed . . . The staff are rushing around.   (Helen)

Ways of working and communicating, for midwives, reflected the ongoing pressures created by linear time constraints and unpredictability. Midwives communicated a striking sense of urgency that led to rushed and disconnected communications. Women disliked receiving inadequate staff time and availability and feeling rushed, as referred to in other studies (Bowes and Domokos 1998; Hoddinott and Pill 2000; Hauck et al. 2002; Hong et al. 2003). Women felt that their needs were relatively insignificant and that to call a busy midwife for a 'trivial' matter was to 'drag her away' from a more important or urgent task:

> I mean, you don't like bothering people because I know that they are SO SO busy. You know, they keep saying buzz us to lift him out of the crib for you, because he's so heavy as well. But I mean . . . you know . . . um . . . it's dragging them away from somebody who has just given birth, or . . . whatever. I just won't . . . I mean something like lifting him out of the crib seems so . . . petty really, to be asking them that.   (Sue – first day post Caesarean section)

As a result of their awareness of the midwives' pressure and busyness, women tended to struggle on quietly, recognising that asking for support or information was to request midwifery time. Under these busy conditions, mothers were reluctant to ask for help, findings that resonate with those of Kirkham and Stapleton (2001b) and Bowes and Domokos (1998). Only some women were able to secure midwives' time, leaving women who were less confident and assertive particularly silent. The more silent women tended to be those from lower socio-economic occupational groups and therefore the inverse care law (Lipsky 1980; Townsend and Davidson 1992) came into operation. Kirkham et al. (2002) also highlighted this social inequality within maternity care settings.

Women made excuses for the midwives and generally recognised the constraints upon them: for example, Louise was highly dissatisfied with the nature of her encounters with midwives but she did not blame them as individuals, rather she highlighted problems with the system and its effect upon midwives making them busy, pressured and stressed:

> I mean it's not their fault, the midwives, they want to give but they just can't. It's not their fault; it's the pressure here; with the best will in the world they can't do it.   (Louise)

Kirkham and Stapleton (2001b) also observed this empathy, expressed by women, towards midwives and they made the powerful statement that 'a number of service users recognised midwives as an oppressed group' (2001b: 147).

Within the institutional settings where I conducted the ethnographies, women's needs for emotional and practical support were largely unmet. Indeed, a significant number of encounters that I observed tended towards the inhibitive nursing actions referred to by Fenwick et al. (2000, 2001). In their research into interactions between nurses and parents in an Australian neonatal unit, they elicited two types of nursing behaviour. The first type was described as 'facilitative nursing action', which involved the use of positive language which expressed care, support and interest in parents, working with the mother, encouraging her, sharing information with her, listening, negotiating, sharing decisions and giving the mother space (Fenwick et al. 2000: 197). Inhibitive nursing action was characterised by nurses establishing their position as expert, maintaining control, directing care, supervising and directing the mother, dismissing women's skills, showing preoccupation with protecting the infant and guarding safety. Women described how this nursing behaviour made them feel defensive and heightened their sense of isolation and separation from their infant and constrained them in their mothering role and relationship with the baby.

Processing the public: the emotional cost

The data from my study illustrate the continuation of the factory ethos within hospitals, with mechanical clock time playing a central role. This has a profound influence upon the ability of health and social care workers to 'care'. Menzies (1960, 1970), several decades ago, described the ways in which the UK hospital nursing system influenced the nurse's emotions and subsequent behaviour. She referred to the anxieties and tensions inherent in linear, time-driven, hospital-based work and resulting 'social defence' techniques. These included task orientation thus limiting relationship building with 'patients' and colleagues, depersonalisation of the individual patient, detachment, denial of the nurse's feelings and avoidance of change. Hochschild (1979) made similar observations of air hostesses, referring to the ways in which social ordering and expectations actually affected what they allowed themselves to think, feel and do.

Lipsky (1980) explored the working practices of public service workers within 'street-level bureaucracies', for example teachers, police and social workers. He argued that the requirements within many public sector organisations made it impossible, within the allocated time, for workers to achieve their ideal conceptions of the job. Therefore, due to the volume of work, restricted resources and unpredictability, they developed methods of mass production that enabled them to process clients through the system most effectively. This inevitably involved the development of strategies to ration and routinise work to alter their expectations of the job. In some cases the workers would stereotype and/or select specific clients who would present them with the opportunity of providing an ideal service, thus ensuring some form of job satisfaction.

Hunter (2004, 2005, 2006) explored the ways in which midwives experience and manage emotion in their work. She studied midwives' 'emotion work' in the hospital setting and compared this with those emotions generated and managed within community settings. She refers to emotion work as the work involved in managing feelings in self and others. Hunter argues that there are several contributory factors to the emotion work of hospital midwives. The most profound source stems from a lack of congruence between beliefs and ideals and the reality of practice within a discipline that has many contradictory values. This creates dissonance between the much advocated low-tech, woman-centred, one-to-one focus and the reality of a medicalised, hierarchical, fragmented form of institutionalised midwifery practised in UK maternity units. The hospital midwife is inevitably bound by the implicit and explicit rules of the organisation and her occupational autonomy is thereby limited. S/he is thus 'with institution' rather than 'with woman' (Hunter 2004: 261).

Hunter (2004, 2005, 2006) highlights the ways in which hospital midwives engage in task orientation and routinisation in an attempt to impose control and keep workloads manageable. They become emotionally gratified by getting through the work, completing tasks and handing over to the next shift, thus providing a sense of completion. To cope with the emotional aspects of work, midwives control and hide their emotions, developing self-protective barriers and boundaries. Thus, to avoid being overwhelmed emotionally, they may enter a disengaged state of withdrawal and distancing. Hunter highlights the effects of emotion work upon encounters between midwives and mothers in hospital and compares these with encounters in the home. In the home the midwife has more occupational autonomy and can undertake a less time-bound, more informal, social and reciprocal way of relating to women.

It is generally recognised that low levels of occupational autonomy accompany working within institutions and are strongly related to occupational stress, with inevitable consequences for service users. Indeed occupational stress is maximised in situations where high pressure, to include linear time constraints, is *combined with* low levels of control/autonomy over working conditions (Brunner 1996; Syme 1996; Tarlov 1996). The relationship between low occupational autonomy and high levels of stress has been identified in midwifery contexts, as has the relationship between inability to experience relationality with women and stress (Sandall 1997; Ball et al. 2002). In contrast, high levels of occupational autonomy and opportunity for relationality with women increase satisfaction and morale in midwifery work (Sandall 1997; Hunter 2004, 2005, 2006).

A combination of low occupational autonomy, ideological dissonance and absence of relationality in midwifery work cannot be separated from the power of linear time upon midwives. Street (1992), in her critical ethnography of nursing, illuminates the tyranny of linear time upon midwives, as my study demonstrates. She refers to the work of Foucault (1977) in stating that 'timetables, whether rigidly imposed or tacitly agreed upon, penetrate the rhythms of the body, disciplining and controlling them' (1992: 109). She discusses the ways in which linear time, rhythms and manoeuvres turn hospital nurses' bodies into efficient machines with activities centring around saving time and using time efficiently. Street (1992) also refers to the stress placed on nurses when trying to make clinical judgements under the pressure of constantly changing and unpredictable scenarios. Varcoe et al. (2003), in their collective nursing ethnographies, also illustrate the continuing nature of the culture of 'efficient processing' (2003: 962) with nurses maintaining a culture in which colleagues are valued for their emotional strength and efficiency. Nurses passively embrace an 'ideology of scarcity' (p. 964) related to inadequacies of staffing, time and money. The notion of efficient use of time is also highlighted in midwifery contexts (Kirkham and Stapleton 2001a; Ball et al. 2002; Stapleton et al. 2002).

This collection of studies, to include my critical ethnographic research, illustrates the complex interrelationship between working against linear time, inability to form meaningful relationships and generation of emotion work. The conceptual lens through which I view my data stems from the contrasting notions of cyclical and linear time referred to earlier (Kahn 1989). As Kahn (1989) asserts, linear time is so deeply embedded within Western culture that any other notion of time is rarely considered. Simonds (2002: 569) refers to the strictures imposed by the medical model's clock, a strict form of linear time, with regard to childbirth and maternity care, and argues for changing conceptualisations of time: 'Time is not only money, as the well-known aphorism claims. It is also power. If we take the time to reconsider these models, perhaps with time, demystification may lead us toward the re-conceptualisation of procreative time and the enhancement of procreative experiences.'

Lynch (2002) likewise comments, within a midwifery context, that 'hospitals are organised as corporate work places overseen by managers whose job is to economise health care and in the case of privatised health care, make a profit' (2002: 180). Within this model, as demand outstrips supply, like other public services, hospitals are always likely to be under-resourced and it is the personal aspect of the service that is usually sacrificed. She observes that we have lost our understanding of the 'rhythm of work and rest', of 'being' as well as 'doing', of recognising the need for 'spaces of contemplation, meditation and mediation' (p. 184). The growing literature that relates to the misery experienced by many midwives working within UK maternity hospitals illustrates this only too vividly (Kirkham and Stapleton 2001b; Ball et al. 2002; Deery 2003, 2005; Dykes 2005a, 2006). Unrelenting pressure upon midwives' time is indeed a key source of oppression.

Restoring rhythms and relationality

A reconceptualisation of caring time is an essential part of any transformative action. There needs to be recognition that carers need time in order to give time to others. This, in turn, requires recognition that caring time is cyclical and rhythmical, allowing for relationality, sociability, mutuality and reciprocity. The political ramifications of the pressures upon midwives' time are enormous and *pressing*. Midwives are currently the main group of health workers and supporters of women during the postnatal period. Therefore, urgent political action is required to radically restructure the current maternity 'system' in the UK to prevent the oppression of midwives and disempowering of women.

A crucial aspect of reorganising the maternity system would necessarily require a restoration of midwife–mother relationality. Relationships are at the centre of human experience (Merleau-Ponty 1962) and these appear to be particularly influential during periods of emotional vulnerability, with new motherhood being a striking example (Ball 1994; Barclay et al. 1997; Fenwick et al. 2000, 2001). In my critical ethnography, the ritualistic, routine, disconnected and managerial approaches of a significant number of midwives reflected, at least in part, their inability to gain any satisfaction through relationships with women. Being under constant pressure of linear time, combined with intense unpredictability, meant that midwives developed satisfaction through completing tasks, getting through the work and going off duty. The women were subjected to superficial, formal, intermittent and time-pressured encounters at a time when they were emotionally vulnerable and lacking in confidence with breastfeeding.

The hospital is a place where women are removed from their community, where medical management is super-valued and rituals and routines thrive. Lock and Gibb (2003) highlight the enormous power of the hospital place over both midwives and women. As they assert, it a place of physical, emotional and spiritual alienation and is therefore counterproductive to independence, confidence and emotional recuperation for women. While hospital may be seen as a place of safety, should something 'go wrong', as Lock and Gibb (1999) argue, it is *not* emotionally safe. The institutional orientation created by hospital settings inevitably reduces relationality and woman-centredness, as demonstrated by others (Kirkham and Stapleton 2001b; Ball et al. 2002; Deery 2003, 2005; Lock and Gibb 2003; Hunter 2004, 2006).

If midwives were able to experience relationality with women they would not only 'give' but also receive emotionally (Hunter 2006; see also Ruth Deery, Chapter 4 of this book). However, it seems unlikely that making small adjustments to the current system of institutionalised postnatal care will achieve much in changing the situation for women.

Conclusion

The metaphor of the factory, with its notions of linear time, production, demand and efficient supply is central to the experiences and work of hospital-based midwives. The postnatal wards form a hub of activity from which staff may be dispensed, at a moment's notice, to other more medicalised areas such as theatre and delivery suite. The combination of temporal pressure, unpredictability and 'rapid turnover' of women make it almost impossible for midwives to establish relationships with women. They cope by gaining satisfaction from rapid processing of work and completion of procedures.

Within the hospital culture midwives are engaged in linear, time-driven, 'productive' activities under considerable emotional pressure in a highly public place, open to many observers. The hospital constitutes a place in which linear time is always in 'short supply', yet reified and randomised, creating challenges for midwives in coping with their daily activities. 'Supplying' for another's needs within a cultural milieu, and indeed macroculture, in which linear temporal pressures are magnified and possibilities for relationality minimised, leads to midwives experiencing their work as 'demanding'. The nature of the encounters between mothers and midwives within hospital reflects the time-driven, rule-bound, institutional orientation of midwives and the ways in which they feel the pressure and cope with chaos.

A radical reappraisal of midwifery practice is needed to enable the forming of meaningful relationships between mothers and midwives at this emotionally vulnerable time for women. We need collective resistance and transformational change to introduce models of postnatal care that enable midwives to engage with women meaningfully, in relationship *and* with sufficient time to do so. This can only be achieved via strong and collective actions through midwifery networks and associated voluntary organisations. If we place the woman and her needs as central, then there is a necessity to adjust notions of time accordingly. This cannot be achieved by token measures, rather it requires authentic and substantial investment in midwifery services within both hospitals and community settings to ensure that establishment of meaningful relationships and caring encounters are given absolute priority. *Now is the time* to proceed with this agenda.

Reflective questions

1   Can you think of examples from your own postnatal practice where you have felt that you have had 'no time to care'? Why did this occur?

2   How can we make changes to maternity services to enable midwives to have 'time to care' during the postnatal period?

3   How can we ensure that meaningful relationships are restored between midwives and postnatal women?

References

Ball, J. A. (1994) *Reactions to Motherhood: The Role of Postnatal Care*, 2nd edn (Cheshire: Books for Midwives Press).

Ball, L., Curtis, P. and Kirkham, M. (2002) *Why Do Midwives Leave?* (London: Royal College of Midwives).

Barclay, L., Everitt, L., Rogan, F., Schmied, V. and Wyllie, A. (1997) Becoming a mother – an analysis of women's experience of early motherhood, *Journal of Advanced Nursing*, 25: 719–28.

Bowes, A. and Domokos, T. M. (1998) Negotiating breastfeeding: Pakistani women, white women and their experiences in hospital and at home, *Sociological Research Online*, 3(3): 1–21.

Brunner, E. (1996) The social and biological basis of cardiovascular disease in office workers. In: D. Blane, E. Brunner and R. Wilkinson (eds), *Health and Social Organisation: Towards a Health Policy for the 21st Century* (London: Routledge), pp. 272–302.

Cipolla, C. M. (1967) *Clocks and Culture, 1300–1700* (London: Collins).

Csordas, T. (1988) The conceptual status of hegemony and critique in medical anthropology, *Medical Anthropology Quarterly*, 2(4): 416–21.

Deery, R. (2003) Engaging with clinical supervision in a community midwifery setting: an action research study. Unpublished PhD, University of Sheffield.

Deery, R. (2005) An action-research study exploring midwives' support needs and the effect of group clinical supervision, *Midwifery*, 21: 161–76.

Dykes, F. (2005a) A critical ethnographic study of encounters between midwives and breastfeeding women on postnatal wards, *Midwifery*, 21: 241–52

Dykes, F. (2005b) 'Supply' and 'demand': breastfeeding as labour, *Social Science and Medicine*, 60(10): 2283–93.

Dykes, F. (2006) *Breastfeeding in Hospital: Midwives, Mothers and the Production Line* (London: Routledge).

Fenwick, J., Barclay, L. and Schmied, V. (2000) Interactions in neonatal nurseries: women's perceptions of nurses and nursing, *Journal of Neonatal Nursing*, 6(6): 197–203.

Fenwick, J., Barclay, L. and Schmied, V. (2001) 'Chatting': an important clinical tool to facilitate mothering in the neonatal nursery, *Journal of Advanced Nursing*, 33(5): 583–93.

Foucault, M. (1977) *Discipline and Punish: The Birth of the Prison* (Harmondsworth: Penguin Books).

Garcia, J., Redshaw, M., Fitzsimmons, B. and Keene, J. (1998) *First Class Delivery: A National Survey of Women's Views of Maternity Care* (Oxon: Audit Commission).

Gray, A. (1993) Health in a world of wealth and poverty. In: A. Gray (ed.), *World Health and Disease* (Buckingham: Open University Press), pp. 81–97.

Hauck, Y. L., Langton, D. and Coyle, K. (2002) The path of determination: exploring the lived experience of breastfeeding difficulties, *Breastfeeding Review*, 10(2): 5–12.

Hochschild, A. R. (1979) Emotion work, feeling rules and social structure, *American Journal of Sociology*, 85(3): 551–75.

Hoddinott, P. and Pill, R. (2000) A qualitative study of women's views about how health professionals communicate about infant feeding, *Health Expectations*, 3: 224–33.

Hong, T. M., Callister, L. C. and Schwartz, R. (2003) First-time mother's views of breastfeeding support from nurses, *American Journal of Maternal and Child Nursing*, 28(1): 10–15.

Hunter, B. (2004) Conflicting ideologies as a source of emotion work in midwifery, *Midwifery*, 20: 261–72.

Hunter, B. (2005) Emotion work and boundary maintenance in hospital-based midwifery, *Midwifery*, 21: 253–66.

Hunter, B. (2006) The importance of reciprocity in relationships between community-based midwives and mothers, *Midwifery*, 22: 308–22.

Kahn, R. P. (1989) Women and time in childbirth and during lactation. In: F. J. Forman and C. Sowton (eds), *Taking Our Time: Feminist Perspectives on Temporality* (Oxford: Pergamon Press), pp. 20–36.

Kirkham, M. (1999) The culture of midwifery in the National Health Service in England, *Journal of Advanced Nursing*, 30(3): 732–9.

Kirkham, M. and Stapleton, H. (2000) Midwives' support needs as childbirth changes, *Journal of Advanced Nursing*, 32(2): 465–72.

Kirkham, M. and Stapleton, H., eds (2001a) *Informed Choice in Maternity Care: An Evaluation of Evidence Based Leaflets* (University of York, York: NHS Centre for Reviews and Dissemination).

Kirkham, M. and Stapleton, H. (2001b) The culture of maternity care. In: M. Kirkham and H. Stapleton (eds), *Informed Choice in Maternity Care: An Evaluation of Evidence-Based Leaflets* (University of York: NHS Centre for Reviews and Dissemination), pp. 137–50.

Kirkham, M., Stapleton, H., Curtis, P. and Thomas, G. (2002) The inverse care law in antenatal midwifery care, *British Journal of Midwifery*, 10(8): 509–13.

Lipsky, M. (1980) *Street-Level Bureaucracy: Dilemmas of the Individual in Public Services* (New York: Russell Sage Foundation).

Lock, L. and Gibb, H. (2003) The power of place, *Midwifery*, 19: 132–9.

Lynch, B. (2002) Care for the caregiver, *Midwifery*, 18: 178–87.

Menzies, I. E. P. (1960) A case-study in the functioning of social systems as a defence against anxiety, *Human Relations*, 13: 95–121.

Menzies, I. E. P. (1970) *The Functioning of Social Systems as a Defence against Anxiety* (London: Tavistock Institute of Human Relations).

Merleau-Ponty, M. (1962) *Phenomenology of Perception* (London: Routledge & Kegan Paul).

Millard, A. (1990) The place of the clock in pediatric advice: rationales, cultural themes, and impediments to breastfeeding, *Social Science and Medicine*, 31(2): 211–21.

Royal College of Midwives (2000) *Life after Birth: Reflections on Postnatal Care* (London: Royal College of Midwives).

Sandall, J. (1997) Midwives' burnout and continuity of care, *British Journal of Midwifery*, 5(2): 106–11.

Simonds, W. (2002) Watching the clock: keeping time during pregnancy, birth and postpartum experiences, *Social Science and Medicine*, 55: 559–70.

Singh, D. and Newburn, M. (2000) *Women's Experiences of Postnatal Care* (London: National Childbirth Trust).

Stapleton, H., Kirkham, M., Curtis, P. and Thomas, G. (2002) Framing information in antenatal care, *British Journal of Midwifery*, 10(4): 197–201.

Street, A. F. (1992) *Inside Nursing: A Critical Ethnography of Clinical Nursing Practice* (Albany, NY: State University of New York Press).

Syme, S. L. (1996) To prevent disease: the need for a new approach. In: D. Blane, E. Brunner and R. Wilkinson (eds), *Health and Social Organisation: Towards a Health Policy for the 21st Century* (London: Routledge), pp. 21–31.

Tarlov, A. (1996) Social determinants of health: the sociobiological translation. In: D. Blane, E. Brunner and R. Wilkinson (eds), *Health and Social Organisation: Towards a Health Policy for the 21st Century* (London: Routledge), pp. 71–93.

Townsend, P. and Davidson, N. (1992) *The Black Report* and Whitehead, M., *The Health Divide* (London: Penguin).

Varcoe, C., Rodney, P. and McCormick, J. (2003) Health care relationships in context: an analysis of three ethnographies, *Qualitative Health Research*, 13(7): 957–73.

6

Midwives, Infant Feeding and Emotional Turmoil

Susan Battersby

The concept of midwives' emotions in relation to infant feeding is an area which is under-reported within the literature although the majority of midwives are women and many of them are mothers (Battersby 2006a). This chapter explores the discourses related to emotions surrounding infant feeding before considering four areas that may present as emotional labour for midwives. These include:

- midwives' personal experiences of breastfeeding;
- dilemmas when supporting breastfeeding;
- the feelings encountered when mothers discontinue breastfeeding;
- 'otherness' whereby midwives absolve themselves from blame and place it on others.

The chapter will conclude by looking at the implications for practice and how midwives could further develop emotion management skills.

Discourse related to emotions and infant feeding

Kitzinger (1998) believes that breastfeeding a baby is a mode of communicating intimately with another human, which involves an expression of loving that often entails intense emotion. Despite this there are limited discourses relating to emotions around infant feeding. Ryan and Grace (2001) found within their study that mothers have emotional knowledge of breastfeeding but that they found it difficult to articulate. A similar finding was presented by Schmied and Barclay (1999), who highlighted that breastfeeding is not just discursively constructed by public and professional dialogue, but that it is also an embodied experience which many women have difficulty in describing. If women have difficulty articulating their experiences, understandably, this may well hinder the development of a discourse related to emotions and breastfeeding.

Discourses related to emotions around bottle feeding are even more limited than those for breastfeeding. In the present pro-breastfeeding climate the experiences of women who choose to bottle feed receives very little consideration. A recent study by Lee and Furedi (2005) demonstrated that there are emotional consequences for mothers who decide to bottle feed their babies. Women in their study reported feeling defensive about bottle feeding and felt they needed to justify its use. This defensiveness is understandable when in England mothers are increasingly urged to breastfeed their babies (UNICEF 1998).

Murphy (2000) postulates that risk and responsibility have become intrinsically linked with infant feeding. The mother is seen as having responsibility for the nurturing of her baby and the mandate to breastfeed is a way in which the 'good mother' is constructed and recognised, in and through, the medico-scientific literature. Those mothers who choose not to breastfeed may feel like second-class citizens. Indeed, some mothers report that they are treated with a mixture of apparent indifference and disapproval by health professionals whilst others felt coerced (Bean 2001).

Research aim and design

The discourse related to the emotions surrounding infant feeding and the midwife has only been scantily explored. Therefore the findings from research I undertook as part of my PhD form the basis for this chapter (Battersby 2006a). The aim of the study was to explore midwives' experiences of infant feeding and was an exploratory research study using a grounded theory approach and personal construct theory. The study involved in-depth interviews with ten midwives and a total survey of 711 midwives in six maternity units with a response rate of 410 (57.7%). The questionnaire used personal constructs to elicit information from the midwives and a space for comments was provided at the end of each set of constructs. This was widely used by the respondents, providing rich qualitative data. The study explored midwives' experiences of breastfeeding both on a personal and a professional level. Six out of ten of the midwives interviewed had attempted to breastfeed their own children. Many of the midwives who had completed the questionnaire also had personal experience of breastfeeding (66.6%), whilst very few

Table 6.1   Method of infant feeding adopted by the midwives completing the questionnaire

	Number	%
Midwives who had breastfed	273	66.6
Midwives who had bottle feed	18	4.4
Midwives who had breast and bottle fed	34	8.3
Midwives who did not have children	84	20.5
Midwives who did not respond	1	0.2
Total	410	100

adopted bottle feeding as their chosen method of infant feeding (4.4%) (see Table 6.1). In order to place the findings from the study in a wider social perspective 37 non-midwife mothers,[1] who had initiated breast-feeding, were interviewed using a semi-structured format.

Infant feeding and emotional labour

Within the study, it was evident that infant feeding and particularly breastfeeding was a highly charged and emotional experience for midwife mothers as well as non-midwife mothers (Battersby 2006a). Four key areas were identified in the study that resulted in emotional labour for midwives. These were: their personal experiences of infant feeding; dilemmas experienced when promoting breastfeeding; when mothers discontinued breastfeeding; 'otherness' which comprised absolving themselves from blame and placing it on others.

Definitions of the key terms in relation to emotion work/emotional labour have been explored by Billie Hunter and Ruth Deery in the introduction to this book. For the purposes of this chapter I refer to emotional labour.

Midwives' personal experiences of breastfeeding

Midwives' personal experience of the emotional labour of breastfeeding has not been explored previously. The feelings experienced by both the midwife mothers and the non-midwife mothers within my study (Battersby 2006a) covered a wide spectrum, as detailed in Figure 6.1. They included positive feelings of enjoyment and pleasure, achievement

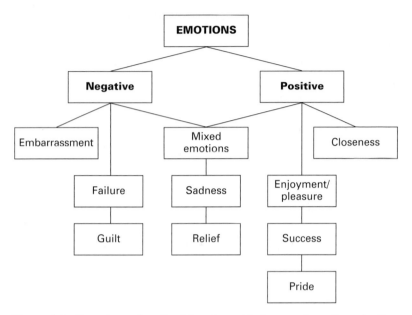

Figure 6.1   Emotions described by the midwives and mothers in the study

and pride through to negative feelings of sadness, failure and guilt. Sometimes there were feelings that fell into neither of these categories and, at other times, there was a mixture of feelings. All of the above feelings are associated with self-conscious emotions which are founded in social relationships in which people not only interact but also assess and pass judgement on themselves and each other (Tangney 1995). These emotions can be either positive or negative. If a mother believes she is successful at breastfeeding this will lead to positive emotions such as feelings of pleasure and pride at achieving her outcome and she will be congratulated by others. Alternatively, if she believes she has been unsuccessful, she may have feelings of sadness and guilt, which are negative emotions and these may be reinforced by condemnation by others.

Positive emotions

Many midwife mothers have positive experiences of breastfeeding and this was evident in my study where 82.5 per cent stated that breastfeeding had been enjoyable. These women described breastfeeding as 'a wonderful experience', 'a fulfilling experience', 'the intimate relation-ship', 'an enjoyment' and 'a great feeling of achievement' (Battersby 2006a). Their words highlighted the intensity of the emotions they experienced and reiterate Kitzinger's (1998) view that breastfeeding is a mode of communication:

> One of the most enjoyable things I have ever done in my life. It's a lovely closeness with your baby.   (MW788[2])

These findings were similar to those in Schmied's (1998) study where some of the mothers spoke of an affiliation with their babies, a unity and connectiveness. Similarly, Leff et al. (1994) highlighted that some of the positive emotions towards breastfeeding felt by mothers in their study included calmness, enjoyment, peacefulness and comfort.

Mixed emotions

Some midwife mothers experienced mixed emotions when breastfeed-ing and it is important to recognise that a woman may experience a range of feelings within one breastfeeding episode. Midwives spoke of both sadness and relief when they discontinued breastfeeding (Battersby 2006a). Often these feelings were intertwined:

> Very mixed feelings. Sad it had finished but relieved in a sense to have my freedom increased. Not guilty because of the good start, but in a sense felt guilty as I did feel a little relieved.   (MW353)

Many midwife mothers spoke of sadness when breastfeeding ceased (70%) and the reasons for this were variable (Battersby 2006a). For some it was the loss of the closeness they had with the baby whilst breastfeed-ing, for others it was because they knew they would never breastfeed again. For some it had been the baby's choice to end breastfeeding and therefore the midwife mother expressed feelings of sadness but not guilt. Even if a midwife mother or a non-midwife mother had enjoyed her breastfeeding experience, some also reported a sense of relief when the experience had concluded. Forty-one midwives (13.5%) described feeling relieved when they had finished breastfeeding and this was not always as a result of problems or discomfort:

> Although I loved breastfeeding I felt quite relieved to get my body back to myself.   (MW511)

This comment reflects the struggle between being a woman and being a mother (Polomeno 1999). The midwife mothers recognised the importance of breastfeeding but there was a conflicting need to return to 'normal' and to be free of the constraints inherent when breastfeeding.

Negative emotions

Frequently when women talk of breastfeeding the focus is often on negative emotions and this was the case for many midwife mothers (Battersby 2006a). Only 9 per cent of midwife mothers stated that they got little or no enjoyment out of breastfeeding, either because of overwhelming tiredness or the pain and discomfort they experienced. However, other midwife mothers frequently talked of experiencing negative emotions as part of their mixed emotions towards infant feeding. Guilt was a major theme and this was not only reflected in their personal experiences but was also commented upon frequently in relation to professional practice. The feeling of guilt was a recurrent theme, with 46 per cent of midwife mothers reporting that they felt guilty discontinuing breastfeeding. This sense of guilt was devastating and some described suffering long-term emotional problems. The sense of failure and feelings of guilt undermined them not only as mothers but also as midwives:

> I lost all confidence as a mother and a midwife when I *failed at the most natural thing in the world.*   (MW69 – mother's emphasis)

> I developed depression and suffered extreme guilt and failure after failing to breastfeed for more than a few weeks.   (MW398)

Palmer and Kemp (1996) believe that the pain midwives suffer because they cannot breastfeed may be worse than that for other mothers. The breastfeeding experience is embedded in the social and cultural world of a woman (Britton 1997) and the ability to breastfeed is often seen as a part of the successful transition to being a 'good mother' (Carter 1995). Therefore, it is understandable that the midwife mother may feel inadequate to help others when she was unable to breastfeed her own baby. She may also feel that she lacks credibility as a midwife when she asks a mother to do something that she was unable to do herself.

Influence of personal experiences on professional practice

It is debatable whether personal experience of breastfeeding assists midwives in their professional role. In this study 89 per cent of midwife-mothers who had breastfed their own babies, thought that it had helped them in their professional practice with only 7 per cent feeling it had made no difference (Battersby 2006a). Some believed the experience had given them a greater understanding of women's concerns, feelings and actions while others reported that it helped them to empathise with, and relate to, women. Personal experiences enabled some midwives to appreciate the pain that can sometimes be associated with breastfeeding.

Palmer and Kemp (1996) have argued that if a midwife has a less than positive breastfeeding experience she can become dismissive or even hostile towards the promotion and support of breastfeeding. However, I identified that conflict between personal experience and professional practice can arise regardless of whether the midwife had a positive or negative breastfeeding experience (Battersby 2006a). Some midwives who had experienced no problems breastfeeding subsequently found it difficult to deal with mothers who did:

> Because I had relatively few problems I suppose I do struggle sometimes with understanding why some people encounter so many problems.   (MW543)

> Because I found breastfeeding so easy, I sometimes feel I have little patience with mums who give up after a few days.   (MW288)

For midwife mothers who encountered difficulties, their feelings of failure were profound and these made caring for breastfeeding women difficult:

> . . . initially returned to work I felt breastfeeding was too difficult and found advising women without being cynical difficult.   (MW21)

Some midwives used their own personal experiences when assisting mothers to breastfeed. This could have positive or negative implications. If used empathetically the mother could feel supported or alternatively she could question the midwife's expertise. One midwife stated that when helping breastfeeding mothers she recalled her own experience, saying:

We are teaching the mums if possible you have to get babies to the breast in the first hour after delivery . . . I look back now and she [her own baby] didn't feed for 24 hours but we successfully breastfed. When she got rid of the mucous, she was fine. So I try to tell other mums this. If they don't want to breastfeed in the first hour it isn't a problem, they can be left because I think for some mums they can get anxieties.   (IMW3[3])

One midwife, who had bottle fed her own children, used her experience to try to reduce a mother's guilt at changing from breast to bottle feeding. The mother recalled the midwife saying, 'look if you can't do it, don't worry. My two have both been bottle-fed and they've been fine' (M34[4]). This links in with the study by Cloherty et al. (2004) who found that some midwives are still offering mothers supplementary bottle feeds as a short-term, pragmatic solution for a mother's tiredness and distress.

Dilemmas experienced when promoting breastfeeding

The second area identified as causing emotional labour and conflict was the health promotion of breastfeeding. Breastfeeding has been increasingly promoted and the breastfeeding initiation rate in England is now 76 per cent (Bolling et al. 2007). However, 24 per cent of new mothers chose to feed their babies with formula milk. The terms 'pressure' and 'bullying' have been increasingly heard in association with promotion of breastfeeding (Battersby 2003) and this has presented a dilemma for midwives and made them wary of promoting breastfeeding (Battersby 2006a).

I feel that women's choice in regards to breastfeeding should be as valued as their choice of pain relief etc. They should not feel pressured into breastfeeding as many women say midwives make them feel.   (MW511)

Lee and Furedi (2005) found in their survey that 50 per cent of mothers reported that they are put under pressure to breastfeed. This was higher than in the survey by Hamlyn et al. (2002) who found only 10 per cent of mothers reported feeling pressured to breastfeed but, of those who did, 76 per cent felt pressured by the midwife.

In my study some midwives expressed the view that by promoting breastfeeding the concept of choice was undermined (Battersby 2006a). One midwife did not discuss breastfeeding at booking because she did not 'want to appear too over-zealous' (MW809) and this was reported by other midwives. Some midwives stated that they were hesitant to inform women fully of the benefits of breastfeeding because of 'the fear of offending women or appearing to be forcing breastfeeding' (MW133). Discussing breastfeeding with a mother who had decided to bottle feed was not perceived as a positive step as it was felt that it might make women hostile towards the midwife or be viewed as coercion.

Midwives have an extensive health promotion role and breastfeeding is highlighted frequently as a key focus for their attention. The World Health Organisation/UNICEF (1989: 27) advocates that 'every effort should be made to protect, promote and support breastfeeding in and through the health services' and midwives in their unique position of caring for pregnant and postnatal women are in an ideal situation to encourage and support breastfeeding. Therefore, it could be argued that midwives could be influential in assisting mothers to choose breastfeeding as their preferred option of infant feeding. This view is endorsed by Robertson (2000: 37), who insists that prenatal educators, which includes midwives, should take 'positive steps to support and encourage women to breastfeed, unequivocally and enthusiastically'. She argues that this is one area where women should not be given a choice.

On the other hand, midwives have been increasingly encouraged to provide 'woman centred care'; a way of working that facilitates choice and control for the woman (Department of Health 1993). This creates a contradiction for midwives, who are expected, on one hand, to provide every woman with the knowledge of the benefits of breastfeeding (WHO/UNICEF 1992) but, on the other hand, to take into account the woman's social and psychological needs (Department of Health 1993). Gould (1996) states that it is understandable that health professionals may be hesitant in promoting breastfeeding because whilst they are expected to provide all women with information of the benefits of breastfeeding, they are also accused of witch hunting and victim blaming when women do not 'conform' and opt to bottle feed.

Midwives' feelings when mothers discontinue breastfeeding

The third area that surfaced as an area for emotional labour was mothers discontinuing breastfeeding. Supporting breastfeeding mothers can be a highly emotive situation (Raphael-Leff 1993) and this was borne out by the midwives in this study (Battersby 2006a). Midwives spoke of their negative feelings when mothers discontinued breastfeeding and these included sadness, disappointment and frustration. The sadness was sometimes because the baby was no longer being breastfed and would lose the benefits of breastfeeding, whilst sometimes it was because the baby was 'missing out on something special'. The midwives reported feeling disappointed especially if the mother had 'really wanted to breastfeed'. Disappointment and frustration were often felt when there had been considerable input and support by the midwife. The feelings experienced were sometimes stronger than just disappointment:

> You feel so disappointed and it's so difficult sometimes, sometimes you feel a bit, I know it sounds awful, but I get angry sometimes. (IMW3)

Conversely, some midwives expressed positive feelings towards the mother's decision to stop breastfeeding, stating that they felt 'happy' or 'relieved'. This was often when the mother or baby were encountering difficulties, if the mother had been willing to try, or if the mother felt happy with her decision. One midwife stated:

> it's the midwives' role to ensure the mother and baby becomes a functioning unit. Mother and family should be happy. If it means bottle-feeding so be it.

Several midwives thought the decision must rest with the mother. For some midwives this caused conflict between their role to promote and support breastfeeding, and supporting a mother in her choice.

Midwives reported not feeling disappointed if mothers had not shown commitment to breastfeeding. However, in this study a lack of commitment by the woman was the main reason perceived by midwives for discontinuation of breastfeeding (Battersby 2006a). On the other hand, the reasons the mothers presented for discontinuing were more complex. It could be argued that one way in which midwives deal with their disappointment when women stop breastfeeding is by distancing themselves from the cause and 'blaming' the mothers. This is similar to the defence mechanisms that some midwives use when they are unable to exert much control over their work situations and therefore look for scapegoats (see Curtis et al. 2003; Deery 2005). Curtis et al. (2003) termed this as 'otherness'.

'Otherness' as emotional labour

'Otherness' or victim blaming is an area that has not been previously addressed as a form of emotional labour. It bridges the sociological theory of emotional labour (Hochschild 1983) and the psychoanalytical analysis of Isabel Menzies Lyth (1988) on social defence systems. When discussing the midwives' feelings when mothers discontinued breast-feeding, I suggested that midwives may distance themselves from the cause by blaming the mother. This is in line with Kelly's (1991) binary thinking with 'me' being a construct and 'other' being the opposing construct. Similar ideas are expressed by Hunter (2005), describing the 'us and them' culture in midwifery that is underpinned by differing ideologies of practice. Midwives absolved themselves from responsibility for discontinuation of breastfeeding by focusing on 'other' midwives' practice. Frequently midwives spoke about how other midwives did not support breastfeeding and identified other midwives as the ones who gave supplementary bottle feeds to babies. There were various suggestions as to which midwives encouraged the giving of such feeds. This links in with Isabel Menzies Lyth's (1988) work where she describes the process of 'collusive social redistribution of responsibility'. When the 'balance of opposing forces in the conflict varies between individuals – some are naturally more responsible than others'.

> Other midwives, I know this sounds really awful but they don't want to be bothered with the time to sit, to sit with the mums and they are quite happy to think 'Oh well, if you want to bottle-feed you go ahead and give it a bottle.'

The issue of blaming other midwives for giving supplementary feeds or being 'anti-breastfeeding' could be classified under 'otherness'. Midwives appear to be absolving themselves for the lack of support breastfeeding women receive or the perpetuation of practices detrimental to breastfeeding by placing the responsibility on 'others'. Curtis et al. (2003) highlighted in their study that the current organisational context of modern maternity care has been fuelling an atomised culture in which many midwives find comfort in 'likeness' and defend themselves against the threat of 'otherness'.

This perspective was evident when midwives described other midwives who they considered were overzealous towards breastfeeding or did not support and promote breastfeeding sufficiently (Battersby 2006a). This was a source of emotional dissonance if midwives with opposing attitudes or philosophies were working together. This links in with Hunter (2004) where conflicting ideologies were identified as a source of emotional labour. This situation could result in horizontal violence occurring between midwives. Therefore 'otherness' may be a coping strategy brought about by conflicting ideologies or it could be a means of managing emotional labour whereby midwives distance themselves emotionally from 'others' views.

Implications for practice

Midwives in this study had developed emotion management skills to assist them with the different areas of emotional labour which included:

- reviewing personal experience;
- protecting the mother from guilt;
- hiding their own feelings;
- distancing and 'blaming'.

The skills adopted can have either positive or negative repercussions on clinical practice.

Reviewing personal experience

Some midwives reported that it was wrong to use their own personal experiences in practice:

> It is important that we don't use personal experience as a bench mark in advice we give to other women. Individual situations and person-alities vary too much.   (MW537)

As a consequence it was proposed by the midwives that a way forward could be reviewing personal experience and considering the effect it had on clinical practice. When midwives reviewed their personal experience they changed the way they communicated with mothers about breast-feeding. Reflection, both in and on practice, has been given a high profile in midwifery education and professional practice (Schon 1983). However, the one area that has not been given this consideration is the importance of reviewing personal experience. In contrast, reviewing personal breast-feeding experiences has been a prerequisite in breastfeeding support organisations for many years. Reviewing is different from reflection or debriefing as it does not necessarily occur as a result of a caring episode or in a structured format, although this could happen. Reviewing personal experience is usually undertaken prior to commencing breastfeeding training or after having a personal or vicarious experience. Crawford (1992) believes that midwives and health visitors could benefit from the self-knowledge and understanding that is gained through this process in order to better support breastfeeding women. A comprehensive model for health professionals to review their personal experiences and perceptions of infant feeding is detailed in Battersby (2006b).

Protecting the mother from guilt

The conflict of roles for the midwife related to the promotion of breast-feeding whilst supporting women's choice led to midwives adopting various strategies. Some informed all mothers of the benefits of breast-feeding regardless of their intentions; some midwives felt it was better to give the information in a low key, relaxed and informal manner; others were hesitant to fully inform the women of the benefits of breastfeeding. Therefore, to comply with the hospital policies they handed out leaflets describing the benefits rather than discussing them with the mothers. This is very similar to the midwives in Cloherty et al.'s (2004) study who reported that they were protecting mothers from guilt when they gave supplementary feeds to babies. It could be argued that it is patronising and disempowering to protect these women from feeling guilty rather than helping them to deal with it. Alternatively, the Royal College of Midwives (2002) questions whose feelings health professionals are trying to protect, the woman's or their own? Within this study the midwives appeared to be focused on the issue of guilt and bottle feeding (Battersby 2006a). Midwives need to consider this issue seriously because the Royal College of Midwives (2002) have iden-tified that there may be cases of litigation in the future which could arise if mothers are not fully informed of the risks and health hazards of bottle feeding.

Hiding their own feelings

Discontinuation of breastfeeding was an area where the management of feelings was particularly evident (Battersby 2006a). When midwives reported feeling disappointed it was important to create a 'publicly observable facial display' by suppressing their feelings in order to prevent them disclosing them to mothers (Hochschild 1983) and creating feelings of guilt. This desire to protect mothers by not showing their personal feelings would benefit from being openly discussed within midwifery. Talking about feelings with the mother may enable them to resolve feelings that otherwise may linger for many years (Ryan and Grace 2001).

Distancing and 'blaming'

Distancing was a way that midwives managed their own feelings. When mothers were unsuccessful at breastfeeding, some midwives distanced themselves from the cause by blaming the mothers. By doing this they were detaching themselves from the mothers' decisions and denying their own feelings (Lyth 1988). They were distancing themselves and cutting off from a situation they could not change by drawing an emotional boundary (see Ruth Deery, Chapter 4). They were using repressive techniques and dealing with emotional labour negatively. A similar process was also employed by midwives to distance themselves when they felt breastfeeding mothers were not being supported adequately or practices detrimental to breastfeeding were being perpetuated. Some of the midwives resorted to 'collusive social redistribution of responsibility', where they split off aspects of their own conscious personality and projected them onto other midwives (Lyth 1988: 56). By doing this they were distancing themselves from the cause of the emotional conflict and blaming midwives with an alternative ideology to their own.

Conclusion

This chapter has drawn on research exploring midwives' experiences of breastfeeding (Battersby 2006a), highlighting that infant feeding can be a source of emotional labour for midwives. Emotional issues related to infant feeding which have not been considered elsewhere have been addressed. Personal experience was recognised as a source of emotional labour and it was suggested that reviewing of personal experiences could be a way forward to help midwives manage their emotions positively. 'Otherness' was also identified as a source of emotional labour whilst 'distancing' was highlighted as a negative means of emotion management. Infant feeding as a source of emotional labour is a relatively new concept and there is still work to be carried out to further develop the concept.

Reflective questions

1   Make a time line by drawing a straight line; place with a mark any positive experiences of infant feeding above the line and any negative experiences below the line. Consider why some of these experiences are positive and why others are negative. Does the positive outweigh the negative or vice versa? Has this had any consequences on your professional practice?

2   Do you consider breastfeeding is important in a developed country? Support this with as many reasons as possible. Do your views coincide with those of your colleagues? If not, why not?

3   What are your views about giving information and support to mothers who wish to bottle feed their babies? Do you feel there is any conflict of interest and how could you deal with this effectively?

Notes

1   That is, mothers who were not midwives.
2   MW refers to a midwife who completed the questionnaire.
3   IMW refers to a midwife who was interviewed.
4   M refers to a mother who was interviewed.

References

Battersby, S. (2003) Breastfeeding and bullying: whose putting the pressure on? In: S. Wickham (ed.), *Midwifery: Best Practice* (Edinburgh: Books for Midwives Press).

Battersby, S. (2006a) Dissonance and competing paradigms in midwives' experiences of breastfeeding. PhD thesis, School of Nursing and Midwifery, Sheffield University, Sheffield.

Battersby, S. (2006b) Exploring attitudes towards infant feeding. In: V. Moran and F. Dykes (eds), *Maternal and Infant Nutrition and Nurture: Controversies and Challenges* (London: Quay Books).

Bean, N. (2001) Is breast always best? *The Practising Midwife*, 4(11): 34–6.

Bolling, K., Grant, C. et al. (2007) *Infant Feeding Survey 2005* (London: The Information Centre).

Britton, C. (1997) Letting it go, letting it flow: women's experiential accounts of the letdown reflex, *Social Science in Health*, 3: 176–87.

Carter, P. (1995) *Feminism, Breasts and Breastfeeding* (Basingstoke: Palgrave Macmillan).

Cloherty, M., Alexander, J. and Holloway, I. (2004) Supplementing breast-fed babies in the UK to protect their mothers from tiredness or distress, *Midwifery*, 20: 194–204.

Crawford, J. (1992) Understanding our own breastfeeding experiences, *The Joint Breastfeeding Initiative Newsletter* 4: 1–2.

Curtis, P., Ball, L. and Kirkham, M. (2003) *Why Do Midwives Leave? Talking to Managers*. Sheffield, University of Sheffield, Women's Informed Childbearing and Health Research Group.

Deery, R. (2005) An action research study exploring midwives' support needs and the effect of group clinical supervision, *Midwifery*, 21(2): 161–76.

Department of Health (1993) *Changing Childbirth: Report of the Expert Maternity Group (Cumberlege Report)* (London: HMSO).

Gould, E. (1996) Don't blame the messenger, *Health Visitor*, 69(9): 351.

Hamlyn, B., Brooker, S., Oleinikova, K. and Wands, S. (2002) *Infant Feeding 2000* (London: TSO).

Hochschild, A. (1983) *The Managed Heart: Commercialization of Human Feeling* (Berkeley, CA: University of California Press).

Hunter, B. (2004) Conflicting ideologies as a source of emotion work in midwifery, *Midwifery*, 20: 261–72.

Hunter, B. (2005) Emotion work and boundary maintenance in hospital-based midwifery, *Midwifery*, 21(3): 253–66.

Kelly, G. (1991) *The Psychology of Personal Constructs*, vol. 1: *Theory and Personality* (London and New York: Routledge).

Kitzinger, S. (1998) Some emotional aspects of breastfeeding, *La Leche League GB News*, 104: 3–5.

Lee, E. and Furedi, F. (2005) *Mothers' Experiences of, and Attitudes to, Using Infant Formula in the Early Months* (Canterbury, School of Social Policy, Sociology and Social Research, University of Kent).

Leff, E. W., Gagne, M. P. and Jefferis, S. C. (1994) Maternal perceptions of successful breastfeeding, *Journal of Human Lactation*, 10(2): 99–104.

Lyth, I. M. (1988) *Containing Anxiety in Institutions* (London: Free Association Books).

Murphy, E. (2000) Risk, responsibility and rhetoric in infant feeding, *Journal of Contemporary Ethnography*, 29(3): 291–325.

Palmer, G. and Kemp, S. (1996) Breastfeeding promotion and the role of the professional midwife. In: S. Murray (ed.), *Baby Friendly, Mother Friendly* (London: Mosby).

Polomeno, V. (1999) Sex and babies: pregnant couples' postnatal sexual concerns, *Journal of Perinatal Education*, 8(4): 9–18.

Raphael-Leff, J. (1993) *Psychological Processes of Childbearing* (London: Chapman & Hall).

Robertson, A. (2000) Breastfeeding confusion, *The Practising Midwife*, 3(1): 36–7.

Royal College of Midwives (2002) *Successful Breastfeeding* (London: Royal College of Midwives).

Ryan, K. and Grace, V. (2001) Medicalization and women's knowledge: the construction of understandings of infant feeding experiences in post-WWII New Zealand, *Health Care for Women International*, 22: 483–500.

Schmied, V. (1998) Blurring the boundaries: breastfeeding as discursive construction and embodied experience. PhD Thesis, Sydney, University of Technology.

Schmied, V. and Barclay, L. (1999) Connection and pleasure, disruption and distress: women's experiences of breastfeeding, *Journal of Human Lactation*, 15(4): 325–34.

Schon, D. (1983) *The Reflective Practitioner* (London: Temple South).

Tangney, J. (1995) Shame and guilt in interpersonal relationships. In: J. Tangney and K. Fischer (eds), *Self-conscious Emotions: The Psychology of Shame, Guilt, Embarrassment, and Pride* (New York: Guilford Press).

UNICEF (1998) *Implementing the Ten Steps to Successful Breastfeeding* (London: UNICEF).

WHO/UNICEF (1989) *Protecting, Promoting and Supporting Breastfeeding: The Special Role of the Maternity Services* (Geneva: WHO).

WHO/UNICEF (1992) *The Global Criteria for the WHO/UNICEF Baby Friendly Hospital Initiative* (Geneva: WHO).

PART II

Emotion Work and Infertility

7

Motherhood Following Successful Infertility Treatment

Helen Allan and Gina Finnerty

Introduction

The aim of this chapter is to highlight the gap in emotional care of women who have had successful assisted conception and to explore the literature relating to women's experiences of successful fertility treatment. We suggest that these are forgotten women, whose experiences in their quest for conception and successful pregnancy are frequently overlooked. It is our intention to put them on the map by encouraging you to consider the emotional aspects of conception and how this influences pregnancy and motherhood.

Helen Allan (1999) suggests that emotions are ignored in fertility practice; we argue in this chapter that midwives and nurses do not explore the story behind conception with women presenting before and after the birth. This story may indeed require emotion work as infertility is a stigmatised condition (Allan 2007). Indeed Kirkham (2007) has argued that much of midwifery concerns caring for women who are 'other' in that their care involves 'dirty work'. Infertile women who have had successful fertility treatment are another example of the hidden dimensions of midwifery due to their heightened emotional needs.

This chapter therefore aims to highlight the gap between existing research evidence and nursing and midwifery practices in caring for women following successful in vitro fertilisation (IVF) and to suggest directions for research. The rate of couples undergoing IVF remained relatively stable during the 1990s, while the success rate of IVF has risen and the risks have fallen (HFEA 2005/2006). Fertility is the second most common reason for women between 18 and 45 years of age to consult their general practitioner (GP) (with the first reason being pregnancy), yet a recent MORI poll of GPs documents their lack of information about fertility treatment clinics (HFEA 2005a, 2005b).

We argue that although the number of couples in the UK experiencing fertility problems has risen, with 1.4 per cent of all births in the UK as the result of infertility treatments (HFEA 2005/2006), there is little research into the experiences of motherhood for women who successfully achieve pregnancy following IVF or GIFT (gamete intrafallopian transfer). Consequently, there is scant evidence for nurses and midwives practising in this area, and British health care staff appear to be unaware of the specific needs of infertile women during pregnancy, birth and early motherhood. Among nurses, Denton (1998) argues that the level of awareness and liaison between gynaecology, fertility nurses and midwives regarding infertility needs to be improved; for example, there are established gaps in services once patients are discharged from fertility clinics. In midwifery, there are no national policies for antenatal booking visits for women following successful fertility treatments. At the policy level, the National Service Framework (NSF) for children, young people and maternity services for England (Department of Health/Department for Education and Skills 2004) does not address this group of women specifically, but does set out, in standard 11, a requirement that women have access to supportive high-quality maternity services designed around their individual needs and those of their babies. We argue for research into the needs of infertile women following successful IVF/GIFT, to address these gaps in the evidence for practice. Our aim is to raise awareness among health care professionals about the needs of this group of women. We acknowledge that, given the demographics and workloads of midwives, adding the emotion work and emotional needs of this group of women could be seen as idealistic. However, anecdotal evidence from midwifery practice suggests that there are emotional costs for these women which urgently need to be addressed, given the increased numbers of babies conceived through IVF and new technologies (Golombok et al. 1996).

Background

The UK's Human Fertilisation and Embryology Authority (HFEA) was given a legal responsibility to license those units providing assisted conception using human gametes, and to consult widely on further policy developments in fertility and embryo research (English 1995). Attempts to regulate such a controversial area have proved difficult, and infertility treatments in particular continue to stimulate social and ethical debate. The HFEA recently published the HFEA *Guide to Infertility and Directory of Clinics*, which provides information for professionals and patients (HFEA 2005/2006). In addition, the recently introduced guidelines on fertility from the National Institute of Clinical Excellence (NICE 2004; Department of Health 2004) for England specify how to define and treat infertility, and outline those patients and treatments eligible for NHS funding. For example, women aged 23–39, and couples who do not already have a child living with them, will be entitled to one free IVF treatment if clinically appropriate. These guidelines are not without their critics (Boling 1995; Lublin 1998; Lavery 2004; Roberts and Franklin 2004), as they are not enforceable and each Primary Care Trust (PCT) and NHS Trust may choose whether to fund cycles of IVF. The HFEA has recently published information for commissioners to improve the evidence for such decision making at a PCT level (HFEA 2005b). Consequently, the inequity in provision of IVF continues. In our opinion, this is a serious omission. Additionally, the guidelines do not address the need to manage the emotional and psychological consequences of infertility and, in particular, do not address the needs of women who have successful conception and delivery of a live birth following IVF.

An underlying concern with IVF, and other infertility treatments that result in live births, has been the potential impact on the parent–child relationship and the child's psychosocial development. Van Balen and Inhorn (1996) suggest four areas of concern with the parent–child relationship in successful IVF parenting:

- IVF infants are seen as 'precious' and parents become overprotective;
- parents have high and unrealistic expectations;
- parents cannot adapt to parenthood after infertility treatments and may experience disappointments; and
- the IVF child is seen as unusual or different by those around him/her.

Van Balen and Inhorn (1996: 4) argue that the majority of studies into the parent–child relationship in couples with IVF children are focused on the development of, and concern for, IVF children. This concern arises exactly from the innovative technological advances that produce ethical concern. They imply that there has been a concern that technologies are 'racing ahead' of society. However, Roberts and Franklin (2004) argue that scientific advances are running abreast of, rather than 'racing ahead' of, society. In our view, this concern should also include knowledge about how women experience successful IVF and their subsequent motherhood, in order to deliver evidence-based nursing and midwifery practice, and how midwifery and nursing students are educated on this sensitive issue. We now go on to review the literature in this area, namely the care of women and their experiences following successful infertility treatments, before evaluating whether this is adequate for nursing and midwifery practice.

Literature review

The literature reviewed in this chapter uses both qualitative and quantitative research approaches. Therefore, we have used the Critical Appraisal Skills Programme (CASP 2003) framework for appraising research. A review of the medical, sociological, psychological and feminist literature was undertaken by the authors. The main areas in the review are: psychosocial development of the child; comparative studies of the experiences of women following successful and unsuccessful fertility treatment and, finally, the outcomes for children born as a result of IVF. All these areas touch on emotional aspects of infertility but do not deal directly with the emotional effects of successful IVF and subsequent motherhood.

The first area of the literature discusses the psychosocial development of the child and the legal frameworks for regulating the creation of new forms of families (Lavery 2004; Haimes 2005). This research focuses on donor families, comparing social and biological parenting, and excludes the effects of successful IVF on pregnancy and motherhood. The main focus of this area of the literature is on how new forms of social and biological parenting affect the parent–child relationship, and how couples and donors make the decision to donate and create new forms of families (West 2005). The literature is from empirical studies of the experiences of couples choosing new forms of reproductive technologies, such as pre-implantation genetic diagnosis (Roberts and Franklin 2004) and egg-sharing (Blyth 2004); from an analysis of the legal frameworks for regulating donor families and pre-implantation genetic diagnosis (Lavery 2004); and a discussion of the expectations society has of reproduction and family life (Haimes 2005). This body of research is relevant for this review, as society's beliefs about what constitutes an 'acceptable' family informs the types of interventions allowed in the UK and, consequently, the IVF experiences and emotions women go through to achieve successful pregnancy.

The second area of the literature focuses on comparative studies into experiences of women following successful infertility treatment (IVF mothers) and women who conceive naturally (non-IVF mothers). Eugster and Vingerhoets (1999) undertook a major review of the research into psychological reactions of women before entering IVF, during IVF treatments, and after both successful and unsuccessful IVF treatment. They argued that, in general, couples who enter IVF programmes are well adjusted, but find the experience of IVF stressful. IVF parents experience more stress during pregnancy compared with non-IVF parents, and IVF mothers self-report a higher quality of parent–child relationship than mothers with naturally conceived children.

In other papers comparing women's experiences of successful and unsuccessful infertility treatment (both IVF and GIFT), Weaver et al. (1993), Leiblum et al. (1998), Malin et al. (2001), Hjelmstedt (2003), McMahon et al. (2003) and Hjelmstedt et al. (2004) make significant contributions to understanding the complex ways in which infertility treatments affect pregnancy, birth and parenthood. Their findings point towards further research into women's experiences following IVF which needs to be undertaken. Weaver et al. (1993) sampled 20 couples who conceived through IVF/GIFT and used questionnaires to measure quality of life, parents' feelings about their babies, and child-rearing attitudes. IVF parents showed no differences from non-IVF parents in respect to marital adjustment and emotional health, but did give higher ratings for their feelings about their babies, and were generally more 'overprotective'. This finding is important, as it suggests that the notion of 'overprotective' behaviour needs to be explored further. Leiblum et al. (1998), using a 'life after IVF' questionnaire to compare childless women (n = 18), IVF mothers (n = 41) and non-IVF mothers (n = 16), found that childless women were significantly less satisfied with their lives than IVF mothers or mothers who conceived naturally. Using a survey questionnaire on 3000 women in Finland (response rate = 74%), Malin et al. (2001) found that women responded well to open-ended and semi-structured questions about their satisfaction with infertility examinations and treatment. The birth of a baby was the most common reason for satisfaction, and the most common reason for dissatisfaction was unsatisfactory encounters with medical staff. Again, this finding needs to be explored to understand how medical encounters were substandard and what could be done to improve them. There is a dearth of literature concerning women's views of encounters with midwives in the maternity services when IVF has been successful.

McMahon et al. (2003) matched groups of IVF parents who had

successfully conceived with those who conceived naturally, for psychosocial adjustment. Their work contributes to a growing body of research that demonstrates normal psychosocial adjustment in parents conceiving through IVF, rather than more positive adjustment that earlier studies claimed to show (Golombok et al. 1996). In Hjelmstedt's (2003) first study, a comparison of 57 IVF mothers and 55 IVF fathers with 43 non-IVF mothers and 39 non-IVF fathers, a measurement scale was used to focus on anxiety during early and late pregnancy. They discovered that IVF mothers had more positive experiences of pregnancy than non-IVF mothers, and that IVF fathers were worried about birth injuries. In a second study, Hjelmstedt et al. (2004) compared IVF parents (mothers = 55; fathers = 53) with non-IVF parents (mothers = 40; fathers = 36), using a self-rating scale to measure parenting stress and marital relationship during pregnancy, and at two and six months after birth. It was found that the inability to conceive continued to affect the current lives of IVF parents; negative feelings related to infertility were not easily overcome. This has implications for provision of a 'space' for women to relate this sensitive information early in the pregnancy so that care can be tailored accordingly.

In the third area of the literature, six papers were retrieved, as they reported research into women's successful experiences after IVF; these were all from outside the UK (van Balen and Inhorn 1996; Goldschmidt and Brahler 2001; Miller 2003; Darwiche et al. 2004; Ulrich et al. 2004). McMahon et al. (2003) proposed that the literature in this field suggests that there may be subtle adjustment difficulties confronting families conceiving after infertility treatment. Sandelowski (1995) made this point some years ago, when she showed that infertile couples found relinquishing the 'infertile' identity difficult, even when they went on to have children through assisted conception or adoption. Goldschmidt and Brahler (2001) assessed the quality of life of infertile couples at the beginning of, and one year after, IVF. Ninety-five couples were asked to complete a life satisfaction questionnaire. In comparison with the general population, both men and women undergoing IVF treatment (that is, before birth) expressed higher life satisfaction, especially in regard to their relationship. Those couples who had experienced miscarriage following IVF conception expressed decreased life satisfaction, and men were more affected than women. Unexpectedly, those who had a live birth expressed no higher life satisfaction than those whose treatment was unsuccessful. Miller (2003) undertook qualitative, in-depth interviews with 17 women who were first-time mothers-to-be, one of whom had had successful IVF. Miller argued that in the transition to motherhood, women's perceptions of the location of expert knowledge changed as the women experienced pregnancy, birth and motherhood. As women became more experienced, so they were able to evaluate experts' knowledge in the context of their experience. While only one woman conceived using IVF, Miller made some useful points about how nurse–patient relationships change over the pregnancy. However, few of these studies have considered the midwife–woman relationship through the pregnancy and birth or the emotional aspects of this experience.

Darwiche et al. (2004) recruited 60 IVF couples who conceived, and interviewed them at the fifth month of pregnancy and at the ninth month after birth. Their hypothesis was that the emotional integration of the history of infertility and the adjustment to pregnancy were linked. Using in-depth qualitative, observational interviews and questionnaires, their results showed that couples who integrated their history of infertility were able to improve psychologically during pregnancy. Couples who did not integrate their history – that is, it was associated with high levels of shame and sadness – were observed to be more anxious and distant with each other. This is consistent with the notion of infertility as a stigmatised condition (Allan 2007). Ulrich et al. (2004) argued that studies of couples following successful IVF treatment focus on the parent–child relationship rather than on the changes that occur between couples. They focused their research on the transition to parenthood using psychodynamic couple interviews, as well as standardised and non-standardised questionnaires. IVF couples had a high level of satisfaction with their relationship, and the pregnancy was described as satisfying, that is, it met their expectations and was free of complaints. The authors were surprised by how 'inconspicuous' the couples' relationships with each other and their children were when compared to non-IVF couples. However, the IVF couples appeared to be less forthcoming during the interviews. As Christie (1998) observed, infertile women are often observed by fertile women (and even researchers) as different and conspicuous.

The last paper to be considered is a review by van Balen and Inhorn (1996) of empirical work that investigated the mental, psychological and physical development of IVF children, and the relationships between parents and children following successful IVF treatment. Van Balen and Inhorn focused on four areas of empirical research: congenital abnormalities; problems with pregnancy and birth, including multiple births and the experience of birth and delivery for the parents; cognitive and motor development of the children, and the parent–child relationships; and psychological development of the children. He concluded that there were no indications of higher frequencies of congenital abnormalities among IVF children, or that their cognitive and motor development was affected. The dangers of multiple births are well known, and transfer of one embryo rather than two is considered to be safer (although van Balen and Inhorn cited less than three). They believe that IVF does not cause any concern for the development of positive parent–child relationships, and felt that the results suggested that IVF mothers 'do a better job in child rearing than fertile mothers'. He also cited McMahon et al. (1995), who found that no dysfunctional parenting styles existed and that there was no evidence that IVF children differed in either cognitive or emotional indices of development. Van Balen and Inhorn stated that the question remains as to whether the effects that have been demonstrated in the literature are related to IVF or to couples' previous experience of infertility. He suggested a tentative conclusion that the experience of infertility had a positive effect on the parent–child relationship. This is also suggested by Golombok et al. (2002) and McMahon et al. (2003).

Discussion

The preceding literature displays largely quantitative data sets. Psychological research on general health and well-being, adjustment to parenting, parenting stress, marital satisfaction, self-esteem, state and trait anxiety, locus of control, reported emotional control, and idealised attitudes to pregnancy and parenthood all suggest positive comparisons between matched groups of infertile women who have conceived after IVF and women who have conceived naturally (a small percentage of studies have also focused on infertile men and couples; Hjelmstedt et al. 2004). However, this body of research has not explored the reasons women give for their more positive experiences following successful IVF. We know that women express positive attitudes in studies using self-rating scales, and from observation data and a small number of semi-structured interviews. We suggest that these instruments and tools are not appropriate to elicit the reality of parenting for these women as they do not explore the meaning over time as women adapt to motherhood following infertility.

For example, in one of the authors' clinical practice sites, practising midwives and a local obstetrician have explained that depression in pregnancy resulting from successful IVF can be severe. Three women had presented at one antenatal clinic in the previous month, one with a twin pregnancy. All were apparently in their forties and required treatment for depression. This anecdotal evidence suggests that the existing research might not encompass women's emotions and the full experience of motherhood following infertility and successful IVF; in this way this evidence from practice challenges research and the reviewed literature. Additionally, data collected in pilot work by the authors with women who have had successful birth following IVF suggests that these women chose who to share their stories with and may never have had the opportunity to disclose their infertility. Indeed one woman described how she had three identities depending on the audience:

> It's more than just having something in common, which is what I have with my antenatal group of friends. But yes, at some point I kind of feel I suppose I should move on, because I'm not going to have any more children and obviously Jake's going to grow up and be a normal little boy, and I'm going to just have to be a normal mum really. Yes, I don't know when you leave that behind. I think I'll always know that I was infertile. I am effectively, because I only managed to conceive with help and that will always be a part of my psyche I suppose, but it's not what I'll probably talk about as much. Probably once he gets beyond his first birthday I suppose I'll get on with it.

The researcher then asked: 'With the midwives looking after you post-labour, did they know?':

> No. I did tell one of them, I think. She then had a long conversation with me about all her friends who had IVF. People really like to talk about it. It's really interesting that there are a lot of people who come out of the woodwork. I don't know, it's strange. Everybody's got an IVF story . . . I still feel like an infertile person, definitely, even though I've had a baby.

This brings us to a theoretical concept: social identity theory, which is implicit in much work concerning emotions and reproduction. Skevington and Baker (1989) purport that identity theory has huge potential as a model with which to examine the consequences of group membership. This is based on the work by Tajfel on social groups in the 1980s. Of relevance to this chapter are thoughts about social identity in the transition to motherhood. Suzanne Skevington asserts that women's experiences are often stereotyped and misrepresented, leaving gaps in knowledge as to what is normative. Support groups for infertile women can provide a powerful forum for representing experience. We are interested in how women move from one identity (being infertile) to another (being pregnant). Our pilot work demonstrates that women who conceive following experiences of infertility find it difficult to disclose their pregnancy and positive experience of IVF with their network and support groups of infertile women. Such networks focus on conceiving rather than life after successful conception, as the following quotes suggest:

> My participation on the [support group] website is tempered now by the fact that I'm lucky and I have got a baby and I have to be careful what I say, and you do feel sometimes that you can't always moan because you're the lucky one. I do feel sometimes, if you do really have a bad day or you're struggling, you kind of feel that you can't say 'I can't handle this.' I mean, all mums find it really hard at the beginning and I know I've been really, really lucky. He's been brilliant actually, but if he hadn't been, I'd have felt bad complaining about it. I'm lucky I've actually got a baby at all.

Another woman in her pilot interview expressed some tension in acknowledging actually being a mother after several years of infertility tests and treatment:

> I wanted to know I was 'normal'. I was told not to worry. But the first twelve weeks [of pregnancy] I was terrified . . . Adjustment after the birth was very difficult. You've got your baby. You should feel grateful all the time . . . Mother's day was very strange. I almost didn't want to acknowledge I was a mother.   (Sarah, with 6-month-old baby following IVF)

These emotive quotes provide just the tip of the iceberg and show that the whole subject of adjusting to being a mother after assisted conception deserves attention from fertility nurses, midwives, doctors, therapists and health visitors.

In conclusion, we do not know what impact the context of pregnancy, birth and early motherhood might have on their experiences, and why it does so. Also, few of the studies address service provision.

Maternity service provision

What are the implications of the findings for service provision? Apart from Miller (2003), who only interviewed one IVF mother, none of these authors considered the implications for nursing and midwifery practice. Given these findings, and the positive attitudes expressed by women who conceive following successful IVF/ GIFT, can we say that their needs are served by current practice of nurses, midwives and fertility nurses? It is clear from this literature review that there is no research in the nursing and midwifery literature, and no evidence of this largely psychological research being applied to practice in the UK. We suggest that this has led to a gap between existing research evidence and nursing and midwifery practices in caring for women following IVF/GIFT. We argue that there is another gap in professional training methods for community, midwifery and fertility staff. We believe there is potential for the provision of evidence-based care to infertile women, their partners and their families. The sort of data we need to identify the needs of infertile women as they experience pregnancy, birth and early motherhood is evident in some of the work reviewed in this paper (see Miller 2003). We need to ask questions that arise from her work, such as: how do women's expectations and information needs change? Who do they identify as experts in their care, and where do they seek expertise?

The relevance of these findings for midwives and fertility nurses are clear: the psychosocial needs of women conceiving using IVF may be different to those of non-IVF women. It would also be useful for practice to understand what makes the IVF parent–child relationship of a higher quality in the context of sharing experiences in the early stages of parenthood. However, anecdotally, few IVF women openly discuss how they conceived; this also needs to be explored to understand their experiences. Understanding how the length of treatment time affects experiences of the parent–child relationship may also be relevant for supporting women during pregnancy, childbirth and early parenthood. We suggest that nurses and midwives have not begun to ask sufficient critical questions regarding the consequences of assisted reproductive technologies, and have presented one area where such questions need to be asked to provide evidence for practice. We further propose that this gap in knowledge base is perpetuated by professional divisions in how the two professions of nursing and midwifery conceptualise care. Perhaps health delivery structures and professional identities have prevented integrated care.

In summary, we offer some implications for your practice

Firstly, more emphasis needs to be placed on history taking and acknowledging women's journeys through conception, pregnancy and birth. It is evident that women need space to express their journey in the midwife–woman encounter and particularly in the antenatal booking visit.

Secondly, midwives and health care professionals need to be aware that these women may be at risk from developing depression both antenatally and postnatally. Tailored support is essential for these women. Additionally, advice for midwives is essential and could be included in the pre-registration curriculum for student midwives.

Lastly, the emotional aspects of assisted conception can have a profound effect on the pregnancy and ensuing mother–baby relationship. As Allan (2007) suggests, it is time to eradicate the stigma attached to infertility and assisted conception.

Reflective questions

1   Given the anecdotal evidence suggesting that the risk of perinatal depression increases after IVF, how can the health professional help women adjust to their new identities as mothers given their previous history of infertility? Is there additional training you may consider undertaking to equip you to help with the emotional needs of these women?

2   How could you assist women to vocalise their feelings about adjusting to motherhood following successful IVF?

3   Reflecting on the women that you've cared for, and having read this chapter, would you approach the care of these women any differently?

Acknowledgements

We would like to thank the women who participated in our pilot interviews and the women we have worked with who have shared their experiences.

References

Allan, H. T. (1999) 'Sister will see you now': Managing emotions in a fertility clinic. Unpublished PhD thesis, University of Manchester.

Allan, H. T. (2007) Experiences of infertility: liminality and the role of the fertility clinic, *Nursing Inquiry*, 14(2): 132–9.

van Balen, F. and Inhorn, M. C. (1996) Development of IVF children *Developmental Review*, 18: 30–46.

Blyth, E. (2004) Patient experience of an 'egg-sharing' programme, *Human Fertility*, 7, 157–62.

Boling, P., ed. (1995) *Expecting Trouble: Surrogacy, Fetal Abuse and New Reproductive Technologies* (Oxford: Westview Press).

CASP (Critical Appraisal Skills Programme) (2003), Milton Keynes Primary Care NHS Trust. Available at: 5http://www.phru.nhs.uk/casp/critical_appraisal_tools.htm4. Accessed 11 May 2006.

Christie, G. (1998) Some socio-cultural and psychological aspects of infertility, *Human Reproduction*, 13: 232–41.

Darwiche, J., Marclay, L., Germond, M. and Guex, P. (2004) Pregnancy after in vitro fertilisation. Poster presented at Annual Meeting of the ESHRE, Berlin, Germany, 27–30 June.

Denton, J. (1998) The nurse's role in treating fertility problems, *Nursing Times*, 92: 87–8.

Department of Health (2004) 2004/009 *New NHS Guidelines on Fertility Treatment*. Available at: 5http://www.nice.org.uk/pdf/CG011pressrelease.pdf4. Accessed 8 February 2007.

Department of Health/Department for Education and Skills (2004) *National Service Framework for Children, Young People and Maternity Services in England* (London: HMSO). Available at: 5http://www.dh.gov.uk/PolicyAndGuidance/HealthAndSocialCareTopics/ChildrenServices/ChildrenServices Information/fs/en4. Accessed 8 February 2007.

English, V. (1995) The role of the Human Fertilisation and Embryology Authority. In: L. Meerabeau and J. Denton (eds), *Infertility Nursing and Caring* (London: Scutari Press) pp. 156–67.

Eugster, A. and Vingerhoets, A. J. J. M. (1999) Psychological aspects of in vitro fertilisation: a review, *Social Science and Medicine*, 48: 575–89.

Goldschmidt, S. and Brahler, E. (2001) Life satisfaction of infertile couples before and after in-vitro fertilisation with regard to the treatment outcome, *Zeitschrift für Klinische Psychologie, Psychiatrie und Psychitherapie*, 49: 197–220.

Golombok, S., Brewaeys, A., Cook, M. T., Giavazzi Guerra, D., Mantovani, A., van Hall, E., Crosignani, P. G. and Dexeus, S. (1996) The European study of assisted reproduction families: family functioning and child development, *Human Reproduction*, 11: 2324–31.

Golombok, S., MacCallum, F., Goodman, E. and Rutter, M. (2002) Families with children conceived by donor insemination: a follow up at age 12, *Child Development*, 73: 952–68.

Haimes, E. (2005) Expectations in reproduction: society and the family, *Human Fertility*, 8: 81–2.

HFEA (Human Fertilisation and Embryology Authority) (2005/2006) *Guide to Infertility and Directory of Clinics 2005/6* (London: Human Fertilisation and Embryology Authority).

HFEA (Human Fertilisation and Embryology Authority) (2005a) GPs say they lack adequate information about fertility services (London: Human Fertilisation and Embryology Authority press release), 20 May.

HFEA (Human Fertilisation and Embryology Authority) (2005b) Infertility and its treatment – a public concern. Parliamentary briefing. Issue 2. Available at: 5http://www.hfea.gov.uk/cps/rde/xchg/SID-3F57D79B-99815583/hfea/hs.xsl/1296.html4. Accessed 8 February 2007.

Hjelmstedt, A. (2003) Patterns of emotional responses to pregnancy, experience of pregnancy and attitudes to parenthood among IVF couples: a longitudinal study, *Journal of Psychosomatic Obstetrics & Gynaecology*, 24: 153–62.

Hjelmstedt, A., Widstrom, A. M., Wramsby, H. and Collins, A. (2004) Emotional adaptation following successful in vitro fertilisation, *Fertility and Sterility*, 81: 1254–64.

Kirkham, M., ed. (2007) *Exploring the Dirty Side of Women's Health* (London: Routledge).

Lavery, S. (2004) Preimplantation genetic diagnosis and the welfare of the child, *Human Fertility*, 7: 295–300.

Leiblum, S. R., Aviv, A. and Hamer, R. (1998) Life after infertility: a long-term investigation of marital and sexual function, *Human Reproduction*, 13: 3569–74.

Lublin, N. (1998) *Pandora's Box: Feminism Confronts Reproductive Technology* (Oxford: Rowman & Littlefield).

Malin, M., Hemmicki, E., Raikkonen, O., Sihvo, S. and Perala, M. L. (2001) What do women want? Women's experiences of infertility treatment, *Social Science & Medicine*, 53: 123–331.

McMahon, C. A., Ungerer, J. A., Beaurepaire, J., Tennant, C. and Saunders, D. (1995) Psychosocial outcomes for parents and children after in vitro fertilisation, *Lancet*, ii: 1392–3.

McMahon, C. A., Gibson, F., Leslie, G., Cohen, J. and Tennant, C. (2003) Parents of in vitro fertilisation children: psychological adjustment, parenting, stress and the influence of subsequent in vitro fertilisation treatment, *Journal of Family Psychology*, 17: 361–9.

Miller, T. (2003) Shifting perceptions of expert knowledge: transition to motherhood, *Human Fertility*, 6: 142–6.

Murray, N. (2005) *Not What I Had in Mind* (Cambridge: Pegasus).

NICE (National Institute of Clinical Excellence) (2004) *2004/009 New NHS Guidelines on Fertility Treatment*. Available at: 5http://www.nice.org.uk/pdf/CG114. Accessed 8 February 2007.

Roberts, C. and Franklin, S. (2004) Experiencing new forms of genetic choice: findings from an ethnographic study of preimplantation genetic diagnosis, *Human Fertility*, 7: 285–94.

Sandelowski, M. (1995) A theory of transition to parenthood of infertile couples, *Research in Nursing and Health*, 18: 123–32.

Skevington, S. and Baker, B. (1989) *The Social Identity of Women* (London: Sage).

Ulrich, D., Gagel, D. E., Hemmerling, A., Pastor, V. S. and Kentenich, H. (2004) Couples becoming parents: something special after IVF? *Journal of Psychosomatic Obstetrics & Gynaecology*, 25: 99–113.

Weaver, S. M., Clifford, E., Gordon, A. G., Hay, A. M. and Robinson, J. (1993) A follow-up study of 'successful' IVF/ GIFT couples: social–emotional well being and adjustment to parenthood, *Journal of Psychosomatic Obstetrics and Gynaecology*, 14 (Suppl.): 5–16.

West, S. (2005) Is honesty still the best policy? Implications for the donor, *Journal of Infertility Counselling*, 12: 26–9.

8

Midwives' Experiences of Personal Pregnancy-related Loss

Chris Bewley

This chapter is based on a study of the experiences of a number of midwives, student midwives and ex-midwives, as they came to terms with various aspects of their reproductive lives. The chapter gives some background to the research and a brief account of the methodology, but concentrates on the findings. It explores participants' relations with clients, and colleagues, discussing findings with some of the most pertinent literature, and offering recommendations for practice.

Background to the study

The ideas for this, and similar studies (Bewley 1995, 2000a, 2000b), arose from my observations of how midwifery colleagues who had experienced pregnancy-related losses interacted with childbearing women, and with colleagues. Pregnancy-related losses in this context included infertility, miscarriage, termination of pregnancy, intrauterine death, stillbirth, or other baby death. I wanted to explore midwives' experiences during everyday contact with women and babies, whilst dealing with their own reproductive circumstances. In the context of this chapter, I want to share some of the findings, which constituted the midwives' 'emotion work'.

Considerable research documents the life-changing experiences related to pregnancy and childbirth, whether it culminates in loss or motherhood (Bartlett 1994; Rogan et al. 1997; Kent 2000). Conversely, there is little available research-based literature on the personal reproductive experiences of midwives, and how these may influence practice and workplace relationships.

Other studies have subsequently been done, for example Rowan's (2003) phenomenological study of midwives without children, which reported the findings from interviews with 15 midwives who did not have children for a variety of reasons. Her findings were similar to my previous studies (Bewley 1995, 2000a, 2000b), and indeed have very similarly entitled themes, suggesting that although the studies were small, the midwives taking part had similar experiences. Rowan's (2003) study also concluded that personal experience of childbirth does not necessarily improve quality of care for women, although in the absence of interviews with clients, this whole area is difficult to substantiate.

Mander (1996) wrote specifically about what she termed voluntarily childless (or child-free) midwives. Her article focused principally on the epidemiological consequence for midwives and the midwifery profession of the increasing number of women who will choose to remain child-free in the United Kingdom. She made some pertinent observations about the probing and personal types of questions that child-free midwives are likely to encounter, which echo the findings of previous writers (Bartlett 1994). She similarly recognised the well-documented negative stereotypes that surround women who choose not to have children, which suggest that they are selfish, and somehow 'abnormal' (Bartlett 1994; Morrell 1994). However, her article was largely speculative, and did not explore in any depth the sequence of events that may lead a woman to describe herself as child-free. Bartlett (1994) interviewed 50 women described as child-free, implying a conscious decision not to have children. However, some described themselves as infertile, and some had miscarried, suggesting that the term 'child-free', with its positive connotations about choice, can be a misnomer. Mander's (1996) work, with its tentative links to midwives without children, is mentioned here as one of the few examples of specific literature on pregnancy as it affects midwives. This general lack of literature on the subject confirmed my decision to conduct a further study.

Aim of the study

The aim of the current study, therefore, was to explore the experiences of midwives who were having problems with any aspect of reproduction, and relate this to their approach and attitude to their work with pregnant and childbearing women and to their colleagues.

Research design and methods

A grounded theory approach was used, which generated written data from 40 narrative accounts, and ten in-depth, follow-up interviews with randomly selected participants. The sample was self-selected, and included female midwives, ex-midwives and students, who responded to a letter in *Midwives* (Bewley 2003a) which gave details of the research and asked interested parties to respond. The sample included those who had experienced miscarriage, termination of pregnancy, infertility (with or without treatment); those who had experienced stillbirth or neonatal death; and those who were not in a relationship where they could have children. The analysis acknowledged the variety of experiences and that there was no one universal response. However, the unifying factor is that of loss, which crosses all the experiences at some level.

Findings and discussion

The grounded theory approach to data collection and analysis (Strauss and Corbin 1998; Sarantakos 1998) established six categories, as shown below. The findings show that some experiences of midwives closely mirror those of non-midwives in similar situations. However, some elements of their experiences relate specifically to being a midwife and these unique elements contribute to the core category. The core category encapsulates the totality of the experiences and is touched by and touches every other category. The core category, and the basis for the title of the research is, therefore, 'Being a midwife who has experienced a personal pregnancy-related loss'.

The six categories were:

1   Nature and impact of the loss.
2   Support, empathy and self-disclosure.
3   Practical and emotional issues around work.
4   Being a midwife, being a woman.
5   Feelings on being part of the research.
6   Impact on practice.

Nature and impact of the loss

The circumstances of each participant's experience was different; however, there were commonalities relating to the concept of loss.

Their emotional responses were also varied, but many described how they felt devastated, hurt and angry, and felt a sense of unfairness at their loss. One said she felt 'a most all-encompassing acute sense of loss and disbelief'.

Others commented that the loss also affected their partners and wider family:

> My family were wonderful – it was their grief too. My parents so wanted this baby too, having witnessed our distress with the infertility.

Indeed the way their loved ones coped had a profound influence on their own ability to come to terms with the loss. After stillbirth, one participant described how she and her husband grieved as if they were on parallel, but never converging pathways. It was only after counselling together that they were able to reconcile themselves to their mutual loss.

The losses also affected their daily lives. One participant, who had a stillborn daughter, then two live children, prior to training as a midwife said:

> Immediately after my loss I went to ground, avoided pregnant women and babies and sought the company of those I felt would be supportive.

Kohner and Henley (1997) reviewed the stories of a wide range of parents who experienced pregnancy-related losses, using letters, other written accounts and interviews. Whilst the uniqueness of each loss is acknowledged, there is a sense of how much bereaved parents have in common. The accounts describe feelings of emptiness, isolation, guilt that they might have contributed to their baby's death, failure and pain. They also describe feelings of jealousy and envy of other women who have had babies. The sight of pregnant women and babies in pushchairs often triggered these feelings, and the thought of pregnant women who smoke, drank or used drugs in pregnancy made many of them feel angry. Moulder (2001) described similar views in relation to women who have experienced miscarriage. These feelings about other women, their pregnancies and their babies were expressed by at least some of the midwives in my study. The difference for the midwives was that they were not always able to remove themselves from the situations. However, some described occasions where, whilst they provided midwifery care, they consciously withdrew emotionally from their clients.

Most literature on pregnancy grief and loss suggests that the negative feelings described above are so frequently reported by bereaved parents as to be considered normal. Indeed the premise of Kohner and Henley's (1997) work is that parents worry that their feelings are abnormal and unnatural, and their book provides evidence that others feel exactly the same. The literature, however, is describing somewhat paradoxical situations. The participants' descriptions of their negative thoughts about other women's pregnancies, criticism of other women's behaviour during pregnancy, and criticism of their subsequent mothering, accompanied by participants' strong yearning for their own lost pregnancy or baby, are simultaneously described in the literature as being both normal and abnormal. In the current study, participants sought to locate themselves and their own experiences to those of others, to assure themselves that what they were feeling was not 'abnormal'. The difficulty for the midwives in the study was that, unlike other women, they were unable to remove themselves from situations in their daily work in which they would encounter pregnant women and babies.

A number of participants experienced depression after their losses, and one said:

> I became severely depressed . . . developed an eating disorder and could not perform my job adequately.

At times this was noticeable to colleagues, as another participant pointed out:

> I said to someone, I think I was a bit depressed . . . and she said 'a *bit* depressed' as if – God, I was awful.

The links between loss, grief and depression are variously described and researched by a number of authors (Cooper and Murray 1998; Wheatley et al. 2003), and postnatal depression has received considerable attention. However, more recent literature (Evans et al. 2001) suggests that 10–20 per cent of pregnant women are depressed antenatally, and that high scores in antenatal depression assessment are predictive of postnatal depression (Hughes et al. 1999). Other researchers examined depression specifically in connection with pregnancy loss, and Chambers and Chan (2004) suggest that that one in five mothers will experience what they term (but without definition) 'prolonged psychological morbidity' after perinatal death. This can be manifested by morbid preoccupation with the baby or fetus, anger directed towards clinical staff or family, self-directed guilt or sense of failure, desperate searches for explanations, and negative feelings towards other babies.

Toedter et al. (2001) developed a Perinatal Bereavement Scale (PBS) to predict those women who would become clinically depressed following miscarriage or perinatal loss. Ritsher and Neugebauer (2002) and Doan and Zimmerman (2003) carried out similar work on the relationships between attachment and subsequent bereavement and loss, suggesting that high scores on the PBS and similar assessment tools are predictive for depression.

Whilst not specifically or consistently linked with a diagnosis of clinical depression, one or more participants in the current study (Bewley 2005) and both my previous studies (Bewley 1995, 2000a, 2000b) mentioned their transient and almost immediately dismissed thoughts of abducting a baby. A small number of participants revealed that they fleetingly thought about taking away a baby they were caring for, but almost immediately realised the grief they would cause to the parents, and the consequences for their professional lives. One, who had had a hysterectomy after miscarriage and other problems, said:

> I cared for a baby once in the nursery who was awaiting social services collecting him. I fantasised about walking out with him ... could I get away with it. I even thought about approaching the Mum and asking if I could have him (I didn't, of course).

Another felt she was discriminated against when she was interviewed for midwifery training, because her baby had been stillborn. She was eventually accepted for midwifery training, but her placement in a Neonatal Intensive Care Unit coincided with the story of a baby abduction in a popular television series. The baby in the series was abducted by a woman who had just lost her own baby, and the participant experienced a series of remarks about baby abductions, and felt she was closely watched and under suspicion. Such thoughts were also mentioned by women who told their stories to Kohner and Henley (1997). Analysis of baby abductions in the United Kingdom and in North America suggests that in abduction by a stranger, the abductor is likely to be female, aged 14–45, overweight, may have a history of miscarriage or other loss of a baby, may have previously 'faked' pregnancy, and may have a peripheral involvement with health services. She may also impersonate a nurse to achieve the abduction. However, there was no evidence of mental illness at the time of the abduction and, in all cases analysed, the babies were returned unharmed within two weeks. There were no cases of abduction by a nurse or midwife (Rabun 1995).

Other participants in the latest study alluded to their fears about disclosing depression, as they also knew of the links between depression and harmful behaviour towards patients/clients by nurses. The cases of Beverly Allitt and Amanda Jenkins, both of whom caused death or significant harm to patients in their care, prompted a much more stringent approach to the recruitment and ongoing occupational health monitoring of nurses and midwives (Clothier 1994; Bullock 1997), with particular emphasis on those suffering from eating disorders, attempted suicide, self-harm, or major personality disorder. Whilst these recommendations were important in safeguarding the public, they led to a climate in which students and practitioners felt unable to disclose the need for counselling or treatment for depression (Dimond 1997) in case their training programmes, or indeed their careers, were placed in jeopardy. However, Brooks (2000) documents her disclosure of depression during her student nurse training, and recounts how appropriate intervention and counselling helped her to recover, and to continue her training successfully.

Support, empathy and self-disclosure

Participants used the word 'support' many times in their narrative accounts, but without defining specifically what constituted support. This was explored further in the interviews, and examples of supportive behaviour included being available to listen, often many times, to the same story, being accepting, not judging, and understanding what the bereaved person was experiencing. There were also those who were described as being intuitive and able to sense when the bereaved person was not feeling well, or was sad. Such people were also capable of anticipating situations which the participants might find upsetting. One participant commented:

> they did not give me a termination lady or a stillbirth lady for several years . . . letting me decide what I could cope with.

Mander (2001) explores support in the midwifery environment, suggesting it comprises four components: emotional, instrumental (practical), informational and giving esteem. She contends that supportive relationships are reciprocal and constitute a social exchange. However, in order to attract and receive support, certain characteristics must be exhibited. In my study this equates with the participants' perception that their conscious or unconscious cues were correctly interpreted by colleagues, who then responded in any of the supportive ways documented. However, some in the study most definitely did not want to disclose their circumstances. Mander (2001) observes that although support is generally considered a 'good thing', well-intentioned but ill-informed actions can be not only unsupportive, but actually damaging. In this study, participants mentioned remarks made by colleagues, for example being told that miscarriage was for the best, as the baby was probably deformed; or suggestions that early miscarriage was more easy to deal with; or that failure to become pregnant after fertility treatment was not too bad, because of the enjoyment of 'trying again'; or that all they needed to become pregnant was to relax or maybe have a good holiday. The remarks were intended to give a positive slant to the loss, but were hurtful. Similarly, the suggestions that participants would be helped by confronting the situations they dreaded, such as caring for women in similar situations to their own, or, for one participant, being asked to care for a woman in the room where her own baby had died, may have been intended as supportive, but were not perceived as such by the participants.

Thus it seemed that support was sometimes consequent on a degree of self-disclosure, with its attendant risks. Some participants found that when they disclosed information they were able to share experiences with midwifery colleagues. Some welcomed hearing the experiences of others, as it reassured them that they were not alone in their thoughts and feelings.

Many of the descriptors used by the participants are also used in connection with counselling terminology, particularly empathy and empathic understanding. All of the participants who availed themselves of counselling spoke highly of the benefits. They valued being able to share their thoughts and feelings without being judged, and said it had helped them come to terms with their losses. Participants who accessed counselling spoke positively of their experiences, but some were unable to access counselling, and some were happy that they did not want counselling.

Practical and emotional issues around work

Some participants found certain areas or certain client groups difficult to relate to. Most significantly, they felt that with the emphasis now placed on supporting bereaved parents, their midwifery colleagues should be able to show greater support for their own colleagues than was evidenced. Participants felt that whilst lay people might be forgiven for making thoughtless remarks, midwives should know better. They also felt that midwives are carers, and need to be cared for themselves. However, there were other participants who valued the sensitive approaches from some of their colleagues, such as being asked where they wanted to work, and being able to change their minds at short notice if a situation became difficult. Clearly, other assumptions were made by staff about how participants should use their own experiences to support others:

> instead of the shift leader asking me how I felt about caring for mothers with problems or pregnancy losses, they would assume that either it was good for me to come to terms with my loss, and that I could not avoid it forever, or limit it to the extent that these mothers would not be discussed in my presence.

Others were also surprised at what they perceived as thoughtless comments from their midwifery colleagues. I had asked if there was anything participants could specifically remember that was helpful:

> I really can't remember anyone saying anything that was helpful. Most people were sympathetic to start with, but trotted out the supposedly helpful statements – you are young, it was for the best etc.

Despite the reported difficulties by the participants, there were many positive comments in the study relating to the personal qualities of individual colleagues and managers who were emotionally and practically supportive. Supportive management strategies around returning to work were key to helping midwives return. Discussions about when and what areas to return to were crucial. Participants commented on how valuable it was to have their wishes taken note of, and how they appreciated being able to change locations according to their feelings. Anticipation of difficult dates and locations on behalf of participants by caring colleagues and managers was also greatly valued. There were some groups of clients and situations which participants found difficult to cope with and sensitive placement helped them to deal with this. Participants wanted to be seen as people with individual needs, not just names on off-duty whose work needed to be covered in their absence.

Midwives returning after pregnancy loss or after diagnosis and/or treatment of infertility may need to concentrate their input to those places where they feel they can function effectively, even if by doing so they cannot fulfil the full role of the midwife. Their sensitive treatment at this time may enable them to remain in the profession, and at some time in the future resume the full role.

Being a midwife, being a woman

As has been seen, the participants shared many of the thoughts and feelings associated with their losses with non-midwives. However, there were some issues which seemed to be consequent on being a midwife as well as being a woman who had experienced a particular set of circumstances. For example, some participants felt they had special treatment, such as being scheduled more quickly for scans, and choosing the doctors or consultant obstetricians they wished to care for them.

While this was seen as good in some ways, there were drawbacks. A participant who had a termination of pregnancy for fetal abnormality said:

> I shouldn't have been rushed, I should have been given some time. The consultant meant well, and was looking after me, and he was going away for the weekend, and in the end he didn't, he stayed around because of me. It would have been better to have left me 'til the Monday to let me have the weekend, to let me have the idea of saying good bye really.

Some also felt that they were expected to know more about their own pregnancies and circumstances, and thus be able to make more informed decisions about future treatment, by virtue of their midwifery knowledge and experience. However, for many, it was simply too difficult to apply logic and knowledge to their own situation. A participant who had rupture of membranes following amniocentesis, and subsequently went on to have a termination of the pregnancy, said:

> I felt I was not given good information, it was assumed that as a midwife I should know.

Similarly, when they returned to the work situation, they sometimes found it difficult to get on with their work when they were confronted every day with the sight and sound of other women's fertility and motherhood:

> I am acting all day pretending to be pleased and happy about patients' 'good news' . . . being a midwife at the moment is making me very stressed because it is highlighting every minute of every day that I am not pregnant . . . there could not be a worse job when trying to conceive – I feel a failure. It is in my face all day long, but I know I have developed good ways of hiding it.

This response was similar to many others, in which the participants talked of hiding their feelings, because their love of midwifery and providing good care to clients was more important to them than their own emotional needs.

The concept of being at work as being 'on stage', with all its attendant stresses, is well documented (Goffman 1974, 1990; Hochschild 1983) and developed by Ruth Deery in Chapter 4 in relation to community midwifery 'performances'. As Smith (1992) observes, some situations challenge the emotions so strongly as to bring about almost complete emotional dissociation, and indeed, some of the participants described how they deliberately closed off their emotions (as described in Billie Hunter's chapter). One said, 'I am surprised none of them [the women she cared for] complained about me being distant and aloof.'

From the findings and the literature, it seemed clear that, as in many professions, midwives adopt a professional face, and they keep hidden from their clients those aspects of their own experiences which may frighten the client, or which may expose the midwife's own raw emotions.

Feelings on being part of the research

The participants were asked why they had chosen to take part in the study, and the responses were varied. Some said they had found a sense of resolution. By writing down their experiences, and trying to convey them to me, as the researcher, they seemed to have explained things to themselves. Many wanted to help others who found themselves in similar situations, and had developed specialist knowledge about certain areas which they were able to pass on. For example, those who had undergone treatment for infertility were able to explain to others the likely side-effects of drugs and the need to have a regular lifestyle. They also wanted to improve practice. They made comments such as:

... anything that can help people in that situation has got to be [good].

and from another:

I feel quite positive in some ways. I think [if] I can help in your research, making colleagues think about how people are dealing with it [pregnancy loss].

Others thanked me for having the opportunity to talk about themselves and their experiences, whether at interview or in the narrative accounts. Some told me things which they said they had not shared with others; for example, one had taken photographs of flowers sent to her following miscarriage, and one had kept a diary about her thoughts and feelings following termination of her pregnancy for foetal abnormality.

Generally, the reasons for participation were positive, and for some provided an opportunity to reach some kind of resolution. One said:

The experience of writing it all down, getting it out helps. I realise a lot of my response is grief.

Literature on memory work suggests that the sharing and writing down of life experiences can help ascribe meaning to them for the writer and for the reader or listener (Browne 2003; Bolton 2000). In midwifery and nursing, reflection is currently a popular method for analysing practice; however, Leaman (2004) stresses that reflection should be carefully facilitated to avoid inappropriate personal disclosure and the sensationalisation of childbirth experiences.

Impact on practice

Almost all respondents agreed that their experiences had affected their midwifery practice. They suggested that they had a greater understanding of the impact of pregnancy loss, and generally thought they were more aware of their colleagues' needs in similar circumstances. Some had implemented practical strategies for their clients, such as forming local support groups, updating literature, and holding annual memorial services for bereaved parents. Others spoke about how they dealt with colleagues who they knew were in similar situations to their own, using their knowledge and experience to try and support colleagues.

Many made a clear distinction between the difficulties associated with being a midwife, with daily exposure to mothers and babies, and the problems of working in an environment where managers and colleagues behaved in what was perceived as an uncaring way:

> Having had a break from midwifery, I feel I have missed it, and the problem is not the job . . . I now feel positive because it was the Trust that let me down, not midwifery.

They felt their experiences helped them to support clients, although they thought carefully about how and which clients they would discuss their experiences with.

Core category

The grounded theory research approach aims to produce a substantive theory, which can be further tested in a wider context. The theory arising from the study, and the core category, is that midwives who experience their own pregnancy-related loss have particular practical and emotional needs which arise as a direct consequence of their work with childbearing women, their babies and families.

Further discussion and some recommendations

This was a qualitative study, using a self-selected, self-reporting group of 40 midwives. Further, this chapter represents less than a tenth of the original study, and therefore cannot provide an entirely convincing rationale for the recommendations. Whilst it is certainly not possible to generalise the findings, within the limitations of the study some recommendations can be made, and some of these may be useful for further studies. Importantly, given the diversity of the experiences reported, the recommendations will not apply in every case. The most important point is to acknowledge the particular and unique needs of the individual. If there is any doubt about a proposed action or statement, consult the person involved about how they feel, and what they would like to happen. This is a guiding principle which applies to all the recommendations.

Conclusion

The study drew extensively on the accounts of a group of midwives who had all experienced a pregnancy-related loss. Many shared their stories with the express intention of improving the experiences of others who might find themselves in the same situation. Others said they found resolution for themselves in writing about their experiences. There have been examples from their stories, and from literature consulted, about unnecessarily harsh and unkind treatment from other midwives. However, throughout, there are examples of warmth and kindness from which lessons can be learned in how to support grieving colleagues. From these examples, recommendations for the future were drawn.

For many of the participants, their losses are ongoing. Some continue with treatment for infertility; some await the allocation of a child for adoption; and for others, the anniversary of their baby's death comes round again. I thank them all for their willingness to share their stories, and share with them the hope that their experiences can help and improve the lives of others in similar situations.

Recommendations

Based on the findings and discussion, therefore, it is recommended that:

- A meeting with the manager should be arranged prior to returning to work to enable appropriate support strategies to be determined for the midwife. This meeting is also important from a supervisory perspective.
- Midwives receiving infertility treatment may need help to plan their work to avoid night duty, and enable them to attend ongoing appointments.
- There should be a clear policy on supporting staff with depression so that it can be disclosed and treated without fear of repercussions on the staff member's job.
- Counselling should be offered, on more than one occasion, and should preferably occur outside the workplace.
- Midwifery education programmes should explore students' own reproductive experiences, and consider how they may affect their care for women.
- Initial and ongoing education for midwives should remind them of the continuing need for sensitivity with clients and with colleagues.

- Support organisations need to consider that midwives and others in similar occupations may need more specific advice on dealing with their particular situation.
- More research is needed to explore how midwives' life experiences have an impact on their care and relationships with clients and their families. Research into support systems, other than supervision, may also be beneficial (see Deery 2005).

Reflective questions

1   How often do you ask your midwifery colleagues if they have children? Why do you ask?

2   What information do you want to obtain from the answer?

3   Would you expect them to answer with more than just 'yes' or 'no'? Why?

References

Bartlett, J. (1994) *Will You Be Mother: Women Who Choose to Say No* (London: Virago).

Bewley, C. (1995) Midwives without children: a phenomenological study of relationships. Unpublished masters dissertation, Royal College of Nursing/ University of Manchester.

Bewley, C. (2000a) Midwives' personal experiences and their relationships with women: midwives who do not have children. In: M. Kirkham (ed.), *The Midwife–Mother Relationship* (Basingstoke: Palgrave Macmillan).

Bewley, C. (2000b) Feelings and experiences of midwives who do not have children about caring for childbearing women, *Midwifery*, 16: 135–44.

Bewley, C. (2003) Letter to editor, *Royal College of Midwives Journal*, 6(2): 86.

Bewley, C. (2005) Midwives' experiences of personal pregnancy related loss. Unpublished PhD thesis, Middlesex University.

Bolton, G. (2000) *The Therapeutic Potential of Creative Writing* (London: Jessica Kingsley).

Brooks, A. (2000) I don't want to cause distress, *Nursing Times*, 96(23): 24.

Browne, J. (2003) Bloody footprints; learning to be 'with woman', *Evidence Based Midwifery*, 1(2): 42–7.

Bullock, R. (1997) (Chair) Report of the Independent Enquiry into major employment and ethical issues arising from the events leading to the trial of Amanda Jenkinson (The Bullock Report), North Nottinghamshire Health Authority.

Chambers, H. M. and Chan, F. Y. (2004) Support for women/families after perinatal death (Cochrane Review). In: *The Cochrane Library Issue 2* (Chichester: John Wiley).

Clothier, C. (1994) (Chair) The Allitt Inquiry: independent enquiry relating to deaths and injuries on the Children's Ward at Grantham and Kestevan General Hospital during February to April 1991 (London: HMSO).

Cooper, P. J. and Murray, L. (1998) Postnatal depression, *British Medical Journal*, 316: 7148, 1884–6.

Deery, R. (2005) An action research study exploring midwives' support needs and the effect of group clinical supervision, *Midwifery*, 21: 61–176.

Dimond, B. (1997) Safe practice or prejudice, *Modern Midwife*, 7(9): 20–2.

Doan, H. McK and Zimmerman, A. (2003) Conceptualising prenatal attachment; toward a multidimensional view, *Journal of Prenatal and Perinatal Psychology and Health*, 18(2): 109–29.

Evans, J., Heron, J. and Francomb, H. (2001) Cohort study of depressed mood during pregnancy and after childbirth, *British Medical Journal*, 323: 7307, 257–60.

Goffman, E. (1974) *Frame Analysis: An Essay on the Organization of Experience* (Boston, MA: Northeastern University Press).

Goffman, E. (1990) *The Presentation of Self in Everyday Life* (Harmondsworth: Penguin; first published in 1959).

Hochschild, A. R. (1983) *The Managed Heart: Commercialisation of Human Feeling* (Berkeley, CA: University of California Press).

Hughes, P. M., Turton, P. and Evans, H. (1999) Stillbirth as a risk factor for depression and anxiety in the subsequent pregnancy; cohort study, *British Medical Journal*, 318: 7200, 1721–4.

Kent, J. (2000) *Social Perspectives on Pregnancy and Childbirth for Midwives, Nurses and the Caring Professions* (Buckingham: Open University Press).

Kohner, N. and Henley, A. (1997) *When a Baby Dies: The Experience of Late Miscarriage, Stillbirth and Neonatal Death* (London: Pandora Press).

Leaman, J. (2004) Sharing stories: what can we learn from such practice? *MIDIRS Midwifery Digest*, 14(1): 13–16.

Mander, R. (1996) The childfree midwife: the significance of personal experience of childbearing, *Midwives*, 109(1302): 186–8.

Mander, R. (2001) *Supportive Care and Midwifery* (Oxford: Blackwell Science).

Morrell, C. M. (1994) *Unwomanly Conduct: The Challenges of Intentional Childlessness* (London: Routledge).

Moulder, C. (2001) *Miscarriage: Women's Experiences and Needs* (London: Routledge).

Rabun, J. (1995) Are there ways to recognize potential infant abductors, and what strategies can prevent abduction? *AWHONN, Voice* 3: 6–9.

Ritsher, J. B. and Neugebauer, R. (2002) Perinatal Grief Scale: distinguishing grief from depression following miscarriage, *Assessment*, 9(1): 31–40.

Rogan, F., Schmied, V., Barclay, L. Everitt, L. and Wyllie, A. (1997) 'Becoming a mother' – developing a new theory of motherhood, *Journal of Advanced Nursing*, 25: 877–85.

Rowan, C. (2003) Midwives without children, *British Journal of Midwifery*, 11(1): 28–33.

Sarantakos, S. (1998) *Social Research*, 2nd edn (Basingstoke: Palgrave Macmillan).

Smith, P. (1992) *The Emotional Labour of Nursing* (Basingstoke: Palgrave Macmillan).

Strauss, A. and Corbin, J. (1998) *Basics of Qualitative Research: Techniques and Procedures for Developing Grounded Theory*, 2nd edn (London: Sage).

Toedter, L. J., Lasker, J. N. and Janssen, H. J. E. M. (2001) International comparison on studies using the perinatal grief scale: a decade of research on pregnancy loss, *Death Studies*, 25: 205–28.

Wheatley, S. L., Brugha, T. S., Shapiro, D. A. and Berryman, J. C. (2003) PATA PATA: Midwives' experiences of facilitating a psychological intervention to identify and treat mild to moderate antenatal and postnatal depression, *MIDIRS Midwifery Digest*, 13(4): 523–30.

9

An Uncertain Future: Infertility and Chlamydial Infection

Hilary Piercy

Introduction

This chapter considers the extent to which women regard an episode of genital chlamydial infection as a threat to their reproductive capabilities and the ways in which they manage the resultant anxieties. This discussion is founded upon the findings from a qualitative research study undertaken in central England, which explored the experiences of women who were diagnosed with genital chlamydial infection and the ways in which they made sense of that experience.

A particular source of anxiety for these women was the extent to which the episode of infection had damaged their reproductive capabilities. Chlamydia is a recognised cause of tubal infertility because the infection can damage the Fallopian tubes. However, at the time of infection it is not possible to identify whether or not damage has occurred and it is unlikely that this information will come to light unless efforts to conceive are unsuccessful.

The theory of uncertainty management provides a framework within which to understand how these women used biological and temporal information in order to interpret their infection experience and make an estimation of tubal damage on the basis of their interpretation. Fertility anxieties present a significant emotional burden for women and the professionals who care for them. These estimations constitute a coping technique through which they managed this emotional burden.

Chlamydia – a threat to fertility

Chlamydia is a bacterial sexually transmitted infection (STI). It is the most commonly diagnosed STI in the Genitourinary Medicine (GUM) clinics of England. The infection is easily treated with antibiotics, which have a high cure rate. However, as it is commonly asymptomatic in both males and females, infection may go undetected for potentially lengthy periods of time. Chlamydial infection can cause a number of serious complications in males and females – including pelvic inflammatory disease, which is a recognised cause of tubal infertility in women.

Over the past ten years, increasing effort has been made to tackle this infection in England. Health promotional activities have been directed towards improving public awareness of the infection; primarily these comprise posters and leaflets which provide key facts about the infection. Three facts dominate this literature: the indiscriminate and asymptomatic nature of infection and the possibility of female infertility as a consequence of infection. Even though chlamydia affects men and women equally, the media portrayal of chlamydia is almost exclusively in terms of the threat that it poses to that most central aspect of female identity. For example, the caption for a recent advertisement which portrays a cartoon female character reads: 'Chlamydia is a sexually transmitted infection that often doesn't have noticeable symptoms and can make you infertile.'

Although the link between infection and infertility has been established in pathological and epidemiological terms, a considerable number of unknowns remain. Tubal damage occurs as a result of pelvic inflammatory disease (PID). PID is estimated to occur subsequent to chlamydial infection in 10–40 per cent of cases (Stamm et al. 1984). However, the diagnosis of PID depends on presentation of symptoms, and a proportion of infection is known to be silent and undiagnosed because it is asymptomatic (Paarvonen and Eggert-Kruse 1999). Therefore, in any individual case it is not possible to determine whether PID has occurred. It is also difficult to determine how long it takes for PID to occur after an initial episode of infection and whether the length of undetected infection increases the chances of developing PID because of the difficulty in determining the length of infection. A final consideration is the relationship between PID and tubal infertility. Women with a history of PID are more likely to have tubal infertility than those with no history or evidence of PID (Westrom 1994) and prompt treatment in those with symptoms appears to be important in reducing the risk of PID and infertility (Hillis et al. 1993). Overall, however, it is not possible to estimate the probability of tubal damage as a result of PID or the probability of infertility as a result of a single episode of infection.

In the literature, infertility is identified as a risk of infection, but in a non-quantifiable way. Risk, the likelihood of adverse effects as a consequence of a specific event (Lupton 1999), is portrayed as a probability. As with all risk appraisals, any calculation can only be made on an aggregate basis and transformation of this information to the level of the individual is difficult (Lauritzen and Sachs 2001). There are fundamental difficulties in attempting to translate the findings of scientific data drawn from study populations to their consequences on an individualistic basis. Risk is the property of the epidemiological population from which it is derived rather than the property of any individual within that population. However, this does not preclude the inevitable question that any individual will ask, and the issue of greatest personal relevance to them, namely the extent to which the data relates to them. In other words, what is the likelihood that they will be infertile as a consequence of an episode of infection? Therefore this is an area which is fraught with uncertainty.

Uncertainty management

Uncertainty is a perceived inability to assign probabilities to outcomes (Penrod 2001). It is recognised as a central component of any illness experience (Babrow and Kline 2000) where a number of components, including unpredictability and lack of information, are considered to underlie the process (McCormick 2002) and contribute to the associated emotional burden. Developments in medical technologies have made it increasingly possible to detect disease at progressively earlier stages and have provided information about the probability of disease development. Consequently, the amount of uncertainty associated with disease development and progression has increased, with a consequent focus on its impact (Brashers 2001; Hedestig et al. 2003; Howell et al. 2003). The rational response to this, to which we are expected to aspire, is reduction of uncertainty (Bradac 2001). Information and the degree of personal control that it affords is commonly cited as the means by which to reduce that uncertainty (Deane and Degner 1998; Eisinger et al. 1999; Lemaire 2004). The required information, an understanding of disease processes and an established cause–effect relationship is, however, rarely available.

Although uncertainty reduction is a desirable outcome for some people in some situations, it is not the only valid approach. Furthermore, the information required to reduce that uncertainty is often not forthcoming: disease processes are rarely understood with certainty and the cause–effect relationships which result in their development are highly complex. Information about this relationship is derived from populations and therefore the information that they provide is rarely applicable in an individualistic and unambiguous way. Uncertainty management provides an alternative approach. This concept might be summarised as the way in which individuals appraise, respond to and behave in relation to an uncertain experience. Whilst it encompasses uncertainty reduction as one possible outcome, it also embraces uncertainty increase and uncertainty maintenance as both legitimate and acceptable (Bradac 2001). It is increasingly recognised as a valid response, particularly in relation to chronic illness (Crigger 1996) and in conditions where treatment or cure is not an option. Uncertainty is important in the emotional management of these situations because it provides opportunity for hope and optimism (Brashers 2001), a form of resistance to the threat of our created narrative of the self (Rose 2000). Information in this context is a tool to manipulate uncertainty in a desired direction, in the ways in which it is presented and interpreted. Such information can be drawn from a number of sources and includes both statistical data and individual cases which are variously used to either reinforce or contradict one another. Thus a poor prognosis in statistical terms may be balanced by a verbal example that presents the exception to the rule (Bradac 2001).

The study

Forty women aged 16–29 years took part in the study: 33 without children and 7 with children (two of these were pregnant at the time of the study). The majority (34) were recruited in the GUM clinic whilst attending in conjunction with an episode of chlamydial infection. A minority (six) were recruited through the town centre family planning clinic serving the same population. Their inclusion provided a longer-term perspective of the experience as their infection was a less recent experience. The women were interviewed in the place of recruitment using a largely unstructured approach. An opening question invited the participant to describe their infection experience. This initiated a wide-ranging discussion within which their understanding of the infection and related anxieties, concerns and experiences were explored. Interviews were fully transcribed and analysed using a constant comparative method in accordance with the principles of grounded theory (Glaser and Strauss 1967; Strauss 1987; Strauss and Corbin 1990).

Concerns about infertility

Female infertility was the one sequela mentioned repeatedly in the data. This is perhaps not surprising given that the dominant social and cultural expectation in Western culture is of women as mothers. Women have traditionally been viewed as reproducers, regardless of their intention or ability to fulfil that function (Shildrik 1997), and it is in these terms that their existence has been justified (Morrell 1994). Their bodies have been socially constructed in terms of reproductive capability and function, viewed as production units in the commodified production of children (Martin 1987). In a society where infertility represents a flawed social identity (Whiteford and Gonzalez 1995; see also Chapter 7 in this book), an infection with the propensity to damage reproductive capability represents a threat to their identity as mother and therefore woman.

Several of the women assumed an inevitable relationship between infection and infertility; on discovering that they had chlamydial infection, they assumed they were infertile. As Julie described, the impact of infection produced a rapid transition from a feeling of invulnerability to one of assuming inevitable consequences, from 'it's not going to happen to me' to 'it really worried me, not being able to have children'.

This is not an unreasonable assumption, given that the link between the two has been portrayed so forcibly in the public information surrounding this infection. The realisation that this infection can be, and indeed is, something that happens to you transports someone from the safety of being uninfected to the danger of being infected. Consequently, they move from being detached from the health information messages to identifying with them. In the process the term 'can cause infertility' is interpreted as 'does cause infertility'.

It was a relief, therefore, to discover that the linkage was not assured; however, the fundamental question, 'Has it caused damage to me?' remained unanswered. This raised two issues for the individual. Firstly there was an imperative to consider the cause-and-effect relationship between infection and infertility and determine the extent of personal risk. This was summarised in the question asked by Isobel and echoed by the majority of the other women:

Is my insides totally clear now or is it a little bit damaged, could it affect me having a child later?

The second and related requirement was to manage the uncertainty that resulted from this situation. The women's uncertainty centred upon the question of whether tubal damage had occurred and the consequent long-term effects, a question to which there is no definitive answer. In the absence of other information, the women created their own estimations of association and constructed their own causal relationships using self-selected markers of longevity and severity.

Sources of information

In constructing their own interpretation of the causal relationship, the women drew upon two key information sources. The first of these was the professional information. In written form this is exemplified by health promotional materials which establish a link between infection and infertility in a vague and non-quantified way. The second was lay information: examples of individuals who had discovered that they were infertile as a result of chlamydial infection contracted some time previously. The women drew on case studies that they had become aware of through personal communication or through the media and identified with them. In doing so they reflected specific anxieties about aspects of their own infection episode:

> On the tele, this woman said that she'd been trying for kids and wasn't able to have any and the doctor had asked her if she'd had chlamydia before and she said no and then when they did tests on her they found out that previously she had had chlamydia and it had gone away on its own and that's what had stopped her from having kids. So I was worrying if anything, if you know how long I've had it for because I didn't really know if it had done anything to me insides, anything like that.   (Liz)

And

> I've read these awful ads, in one of my magazines that I read, and this lady, she got pains in her stomach, she thought she was pregnant and she was only 15 and she'd actually got chlamydia and now she's had a hysterectomy, she can't have kids and she's 15 years old. (Jodie)

The diagnosis of an STI is rarely shared with others because of the social stigma associated with these infections. Consequently these accounts exist in a relative vacuum of social discourse and are therefore accorded disproportionate significance; few people will know of others who have had the infection and subsequently conceived without difficulty. The personal and emotive nature of the accounts makes them particularly powerful and memorable, all the more so because they are largely unchallenged. Additional perceived similarities between self and the subject of the account served to further strengthen the conviction that the infection had caused long-term damage as Kelly explained:

> I am worried because my neighbour next door, she can't have any children anymore and the reason for that is that she's had chlamydia as well, and when she had her first baby, her little lad, she went down to 6 stone and she went to the hospital and they tested her and she had chlamydia and I've lost quite a lot of weight rapidly, it's just dropped. Chlamydia doesn't really have anything to do with your weight but it's funny how she lost quite a bit of weight and so have I and we've both had the same disease.   (Kelly)

The women linked their assumptions about the probability of tubal damage to two factors, namely the duration of infection and the severity of symptoms. These concepts were employed either independently of one another or in conjunction with one another. The underlying assumption in both respects was of a direct proportional relationship between cause and effect. Effectively, it was assumed that the more severe the symptoms, the greater the probability that damage had occurred. Similarly, the longer the estimated period of infection, the greater the probability of tubal damage.

The question, however, remains: what duration of infectivity and what degree of severity were assumed to cause damage and what constituted the knowledge base upon which these estimations were made? Although there was an implied objectivity in this causal relationship, the absence of any empirical data necessitated the objectification of subjective information, assessments and interpretations. For a few women it was simply common sense: an infection that had been present for only a few weeks was unlikely to cause damage. In most cases, however, it was evident that the women made personal assessments against the benchmark of information available to them, particularly lay sources of information.

Duration as an indication of damage

It was assumed that the longer the infection had been present, the greater the probability that it may have caused damage. This would appear to be a reasonable assumption although there are no data to support it. However, it does not address the central question – how long does an infection have to be present for it to cause damage such that it affects fertility? The working principle adopted by those women who assumed they had escaped damage was that the length of time that it takes for damage to occur is greater than the estimated length of their infection, whether this was weeks, months or years. This was the basis upon which Shirley made her estimation of risk:

> I just assume that because I could only have had it for a few weeks sort of thing that it can't really have done much damage but I don't know, whether these things can do much damage in a couple of weeks, I just assume that it didn't.   (Shirley)

Several respondents referred to the possibility that someone could have the infection for a long time and be unaware of the fact, often until they attempted to conceive. A range of information sources were quoted to support such explanations, including media reports and the experiences of friends and acquaintances. However, although they acknowledged that the infection was characterised by an asymptomatic stage, the underpinning assumption was that symptoms would occur at some point, that the infection would eventually become manifest albeit after a largely unspecified but possibly lengthy period of time. In this respect symptoms were viewed positively, particularly if they occurred sooner than expected, as Jane explained:

> I know when I've read leaflets that it says women can carry it for years without having any symptoms at all, well for a long time anyway, but I know that I hadn't had it that long and so I really didn't expect to get the symptoms as soon as I'd got them, I mean I'm glad that I had because I, now I've found out that I've got it but . . .   (Jane)

The appearance of symptoms enabled detection and treatment, thereby shortening the duration of infection and the consequent implications. However, complacency about the probability of having escaped tubal damage was tempered by concerns that symptomatic presentation may not have occurred in time to enable treatment prior to the occurrence of damage:

> It might not flare up for 5 years and it's too late then, before you know. (Paula)

Severity as an indication of damage

An alternative interpretation of symptoms was as an indication of damage having occurred. The women had experienced a range of symptoms which they attributed to the infection. However, the linkage with severity was confined to one specific symptom, namely the level of pain experienced. This was interpreted either as a direct indication of damage or as an indication of duration of infection which was in turn associated with damage. For Liz, the level of pain equated directly to concerns of infertility:

> That [infertility] did worry me especially like with the pain that I was having.

Jane made the same linkage, although as this was the second episode of infection, she had opportunity to compare experiences. Subsequent to her first episode, which was asymptomatic, she became pregnant, thereby confirming tubal patency. On this basis the severe pain associated with her second episode of infection was a matter of particular concern:

> I know from the time before when I had it that it didn't leave me infertile because I did get pregnant, but this time because of the severe pains that I've had in my tubes, it worries me more this time than it did last time.

Julie, who did not know how long she had been infected but had experienced severe symptoms, sufficient to merit hospitalisation, assumed a threefold linkage. She linked severity and longevity on the basis of her own experience:

> Obviously if I was in that much pain it could probably have been there for a while . . . the pain that I've had, is it because I've had it a long time?

Thirdly, she constructed a link between longevity and infertility on the basis of anecdotal information:

> It really worried me, not being able to have children, it really did . . . because my mum said, 'Oh, this woman's been on the telly, she's had it for 12 years and she can't have children.'

These factors provided the basis of a retrospective assessment of the damage caused by infection. However, they were used as the basis of two oppositional constructions. For those who considered that they had had a long and/or severe infection, they formed the basis of anxieties surrounding infertility, whilst for those who considered themselves to have had a short or mild infection they were used as a means of relieving anxiety.

Catching it in time

A number of the respondents equated the value of diagnosis with the opportunity to receive treatment and eliminate the infection. Several described this as 'catching it in time', the implication being that the treatment and cure served as a safeguard against tubal damage:

> I'm glad that I'm getting it treated and not to leave it because if not I would be infertile . . . in time to come if I ever want children if I don't have it treated I'll not be able to have any.   (Kate)

Treatment provided the means by which to protect oneself from damage, in contrast to those case studies portrayed in the media: the women who had not been afforded this opportunity with the apparently inevitable consequences of not being treated. This perspective focused on the potential damage prevented as a result of treatment rather than on the unquantifiable and unalterable damage that may already have occurred. It represents positive action, a means by which to manage uncertainty through reclaiming control and re-establishing the predictability of a body-self threatened by the presence of infection (Frank 1995).

The professional perspective

When confronted by the diagnosis of infection and the consequent uncertainties surrounding infertility, asking questions and seeking information constitutes a response to that uncertainty. The health professionals who are concerned with treatment and management of the infection have an essential role as a source of information and support for those emotionally traumatised by the infection experience (Piercy 2006). They also represent a safe and expert potential source of knowledge. Several of the respondents sought a definitive test that could provide unequivocal information:

> I did ask them when I came last time, I said is there anything that can, any way that you know [that I can become pregnant], and they said no, you can't test for it can you? (Michelle)

This reflects a mechanistic paradigm of medicine in which diagnostic testing is the link between cause and effect. However, in this situation there are no technological procedures available to provide such information, no tests that can unequivocally resolve the uncertain issue of fertility. The only way that someone can definitively determine their fertility is by becoming pregnant. This leaves medical opinion as the only source of information on this matter, an opinion which occupies a largely unquestioned position of dominance by drawing upon both common sense and technical explanatory models (Oakley 1984).

Communication of risk

The communication of risk on an individual basis is a common aspect of medical practice; however, it is intrinsically problematic. A discussion of percentage probabilities that relates to a group of people has little relevance for the individual who wants to know specifically about their own life chances. People are generally considered to apply a bimodal model of risk in which they see themselves as either high or low risk, which bears little relevance to the mathematical models used by doctors (Misselbrook and Armstrong 2002). In communicating risk, the challenge is to provide understandable information that has personal relevance and reflects the probable health effect in a comprehensible form.

Whilst the way that information is presented is highly relevant in this respect, arguably the way that it is received is of greater concern. The specific terminology and approach of the health professionals are important. However, an individual's beliefs influence how they interpret health messages and assimilate them into a wider understanding of the infection. It is the 'take home message' that they glean from that consultation, and the extent to which it either reinforces or extends their own interpretation of the situation, which is of particular relevance in this respect.

The respondents reported a health professional viewpoint that largely mirrored their own although with an emphasis on the importance of treating and eliminating infection. In answer to the central question 'am I infertile?', all the respondents reported a non-committal response that neither confirmed nor rejected the possibility. The question of fertility and conception was one for the future, to be answered at some later, indefinite time:

> she told me just to forget about it for now because what worried me the most was when later on, if I want to have children and that's the one thing that's really worrying me, but she said just to forget about it and when the time comes and you want to try, she said you'll just have to keep trying, that's what worried me the most.   (Jacky)

In several accounts, the way that the health professionals' viewpoints were recounted suggests that they were largely optimistic, suggestive of a favourable outcome. The health professional can be no more confident than the patient that damage has not occurred. Whilst such a stance may be simply pragmatic on the basis that statistically the majority of women will not have problems, it could also serve as a coping strategy by which health professionals protect themselves from the emotionally laden situation of a patient confronting possible bad news. However, if this professional judgement does not appear to take into account unanswered questions, such as the duration of a particular infection episode, its impact upon the emotional burden of the woman is questionable:

> I just said, I said to her that I'd heard it could stop you having children and she said oh that's only if it's gone on for a very long time but I didn't know how long I'd had it for or anything.   (Liz)

Distancing the problem

Although women made their own assessments of damage or sought information from health professionals, they did recognise that ultimately they had no means by which to obtain definitive information. This effectively limited their ability to reduce uncertainty. Distancing themselves in temporal terms enabled them to manage the continued uncertainty. In so far as pregnancy was a matter for the future, so too were the potential problems associated with it. The most common response, as summarised by Jill, was to wait and see, to deal with the matter as and when it occurred:

> I suppose the major thing was, you know, I hope I don't become sterile, but again, as I've said I'm not going to know for another 10 years and so it's a waste of energy to worry about stuff like that now.

However, when that time does come the uncertainties around fertility may well re-emerge and cause considerable anxieties, particularly if women have unrealistic expectations about the length of time that it may take to conceive, as Jane identified:

> I know if I think we'll try for a baby, I know roughly when and if I don't get caught then I think first month I'll panic and second month I'll panic even more and the third month I don't know what I'll do.

When respondents did reflect on the possibility of future fertility problems, the New Reproductive Technologies (NRTs) were envisaged as a solution to their potential problem. The proliferation of these technologies represents a medical, industrialised approach to the problem of infertility where new techniques reconstruct an unachievable pregnancy as a not-yet-achieved pregnancy. Although this belies the reality that for many this is beset by unattainability, enormous personal cost and frequent failure, the image of endless possibilities is portrayed in the media, which reinforces the authority of biomedicine (Whiteford and Gonzalez 1995). It is unsurprising, therefore, that respondents identified NRT as the solution, a means by which to overcome the uncertainty of infertility. NRT offers a means by which to fulfil the social desire to have a child, a way in which to bypass infertility (Shildrik 1997). Reproduction in these terms is a technological process, produced and sanctioned by the authoritative knowledge of biomedicine. NRTs offer a degree of control over those life choices and cultural expectations that are threatened by a susceptible and potentially damaged body. If technology cannot provide definitive answers at present to the central question of fertility, it does promise a resolution to the uncertainty that chlamydial infection creates by bypassing the problem of infertility.

Conclusion

Concerns about fertility are a source of considerable anxiety for women diagnosed with chlamydial infection. These anxieties are reflected in and reinforced through the health promotion literature, which presents a view of women defined in terms of their reproductive capabilities. In the absence of definitive information, women draw on a range of physical indicators and social comparisons and use them as information sources in order to try and reduce their resultant uncertainty. These pieces of information provide benchmarks against which they estimate the likelihood of tubal damage. Assessments of severity and duration of infection are particularly significant in this respect. Pain is commonly taken as an indication of both severity and duration and is therefore viewed as considerably more sinister than other symptoms. These indicators are used in a similar way by health professionals.

These techniques appear to be effective in reducing the anxieties associated with infertility that occur around the time of infection. However, their effectiveness is inevitably limited and may well be challenged when circumstances change and women attempt to conceive. An alternative approach was to accept continued uncertainty and reduce current anxieties by postponing any fertility considerations, although anxieties may well re-emerge when women attempt to conceive.

The number of women diagnosed with chlamydial infection will continue to increase as a result of increasing incidence rates and increased testing and screening activity. Consequently the number of women who are required to face uncertainties about their fertility will also increase. Implementation of a national screening programme in England (Department of Health 2001) will result in increased detection of asymptomatic infection. The extent to which this will have an impact on fertility anxieties is a matter for speculation. Overall, however, the collective emotional burden on women, and those health professionals who support and care for them, seems set to increase and should not be underestimated. The ramifications of these anxieties are likely to extend well beyond initial diagnosis and treatment of infection and may affect women throughout the rest of their reproductive lifespan.

Reflective questions

1   To what extent do you consider that health promotional messages which link chlamydia to infertility have an effect upon sexual behaviour, initiating health protective behaviours?

2   In what ways might women's fertility anxieties, subsequent to chlamydial infection, influence their contraception and conception behaviours?

3   Consider how this may affect their use of sexual health service provision.

References

Babrow, A. and Kline, K. (2000) From 'reducing' to 'coping with' uncertainty: reconceptualizing the central challenge in breast self-exams, *Social Science and Medicine*, 51: 1805–16.

Bradac, J. (2001) Theory comparison: uncertainty reduction, problematic integration, uncertainty management and other curious constructs, *Journal of Communication*, 51(3): 456–76.

Brashers, D. (2001) Communication and uncertainty management, *Journal of Communication*, 51(3): 477–97.

Crigger, N. (1996) Testing an uncertainty model for women with multiple sclerosis, *Advances in Nursing Science*, 18(3): 37–47.

Deane, K. and Degner, L. (1998) Information needs, uncertainty and anxiety in women who had a breast biopsy with benign outcome, *Cancer Nursing*, 21(2): 117–26.

Department of Health (2001) *Sexual Health and HIV Strategy* (London: Department of Health).

Eisinger, F., Geller, G., Burke, W. and Holtzman, N. A. (1999) Cultural basis for differences between US and French clinical recommendations for women at increased risk of breast and ovarian cancer, *The Lancet*, 353: 919–20.

Frank, A. (1995) *The Wounded Storyteller: Body, Illness and Ethics* (Chicago: University of Chicago Press).

Glaser, B. and Strauss, A. (1967) *The Discovery of Grounded Theory: Strategies for Qualitative Research* (New York: Aldine de Gruyter).

Hedestig, O., Sandman, P. and Widmark, A. (2003) Living with untreated localized prostate cancer: a qualitative analysis of patient narratives, *Cancer Nursing*, 26(1): 55–60.

Hillis, S., Coles, B., Litchfield, B., Black, C., Mojica, B., Schmidt, K. and St Louis, M. (1993) Delayed care of pelvic inflammatory disease as a risk factor for impaired fertility, *American Journal of Obstetrics and Gynaecology*, 168: 1503–9.

Howell, D., Fitch, D. and Deane, K. (2003) Impact of ovarian cancer perceived by women, *Cancer Nursing* 26(1): 1–9.

Lauritzen, S. and Sachs, L. (2001) Normality, risks and the future: implicit communication of threat in health surveillance, *Sociology of Health and Illness*, 23(4): 497–516.

Lemaire, J. (2004) More than just menstrual cramps: symptoms and uncertainty among women with endometriosis, *Journal of Obstetric Gynaecological and Neonatal Nursing*, 3(1): 71–9.

Lupton, D. (1999) Introduction: risk and sociocultural theory. In: D. Lupton, *Risk and Sociocultural Theory: New Directions and Perspectives* (Cambridge: Cambridge University Press).

Martin, E. (1987) *The Woman in the Body* (Buckingham: Open University Press).

McCormick, K. (2002) A concept analysis of uncertainty in illness, *Journal of Nursing Scholarship*, 34(2): 127–31.

Misselbrook, D. and Armstrong, D. (2002) Thinking about risk: can doctors and patients talk the same language? *Family Practice*, 19(1): 1–2.

Morrell, C. (1994) *Unwomanly Conduct: The Challenges of Intentional Childlessness* (New York: Routledge).

Oakley, A. (1984) *The Captured Womb: A History of the Medical Care of Pregnant Women* (Oxford: Blackwell).

Paarvonen, J. and Eggert-Kruse, W. (1999) Chlamydia trachomatis: impact on human reproduction, *Human Reproduction Update*, 5(5): 433–47.

Penrod, J. (2001) Refinement of the concept of uncertainty. *Journal of Advanced Nursing*, 34(2): 238–45.

Piercy, H. (2006) The importance of contextualisation in giving a diagnosis of genital chlamydial infection: findings from a qualitative study, *Journal of Family Planning and Reproductive Health Care*, 32(4): 227–30.

Rose, H. (2000) Risk, trust and scepticism in the age of new genetics. In: B. Adam, U. Beck and J. V. Loon (eds), *The Risk Society and Beyond* (London: Sage).

Shildrik, M. (1997) *Leaky Bodies and Boundaries: Feminism, Postmodernism and (Bio)ethics* (New York: Routledge).

Stamm, W., Guinan, M., Johnson, C., Starcher, T., King, H. and McCormack, W. (1984) Effect of treatment regimens for *Neisseria gonorrhoeae* on simultaneous infection with *Chlamydia trachomatis*, *New England Journal of Medicine*, 310: 545–9.

Strauss, A. (1987) *Qualitative Analysis for Social Scientists* (Cambridge: Cambridge University Press).

Strauss, A. and Corbin, J. (1990) *Basics of Qualitative Research: Grounded Theory Procedures and Techniques* (Newbury Park, CA: Sage).

Westrom, L. (1994) Sexually transmitted diseases and infertility, *Sexually Transmitted Infections*, 21: S32–7.

Whiteford, L. and Gonzalez, L. (1995) Stigma: the hidden burden of infertility, *Social Science and Medicine*, 40(1): 27–36.

PART III

Developing Emotional Awareness in Health Care Practitioners

10

'Mixed Messages': Midwives' Experiences of Managing Emotion

Billie Hunter

Introduction

This chapter explores how midwives manage their emotions, focusing particularly on the experiences of 'novice' midwives (that is, student midwives and those in their first year of qualification). It draws on findings from my doctoral research study, which was supported by an Iolanthe Midwifery Trust Research Fellowship between 1999 and 2001 and which explored how student and qualified midwives experienced and managed emotions at work (Hunter 2002). The findings related to sources of emotion work have been discussed elsewhere (Hunter 2004, 2005, 2006). This chapter focuses on how emotions are managed. Using illustrations from midwives' accounts and fieldwork observations, I will explore how the skills of emotion management are learnt, and identify both the feeling rules that inform emotional display and the various strategies that midwives employ to manage their emotions. There appeared to be an emotion management continuum, with, at one end, suppression of emotion ('affective neutrality'), and, at the other, expression of emotion ('affective awareness').

I will describe how these differing approaches to managing emotion were manifested in midwives' behaviour and affected novices' experiences. The chapter begins with a brief overview of the research study, before discussing in detail these approaches and their effects.

Research study

The research study was conducted between 1997 and 2002, in an area of South Wales. An ethnographic approach was used, and data were collected via focus groups, participant observation and interviews, in order to gain as many insights as possible.

Student midwives from both 18-month and three-year educational programmes took part in four focus groups (n = 27). Forty qualified midwives participated in focus groups, workplace observations and interviews. Purposive sampling was used to ensure that participants represented a variety of clinical contexts, levels of clinical responsibility and lengths of experience. With permission, interviews and focus groups were audio-taped and transcribed verbatim; detailed field notes were taken during the periods of observation. All data were thematically analysed.[1]

The overall aim of the study was to explore how midwives experienced and managed emotion at work. I was interested in exploring how this was affected by the clinical context in which the midwife worked, level of clinical responsibility, and whether the experiences of student and qualified midwives differed.

Learning to manage emotion: mixed messages

Midwifery was generally experienced as highly emotional work, thus an important part of the occupational socialisation process was learning to deal with the intensity of these emotions. Students learnt 'what midwives do' in relation to emotional display through trial and error. As Smith (1992) found in her study of student nurse socialisation, the information regarding emotion display was subtle. Students appeared to 'pick up' the rules from a variety of sources: for example, by observing the behaviour of other midwives, from verbal and non-verbal interactions with senior midwives and during peer group discussions. It was rare to find that emotional issues had been addressed overtly; more commonly, the 'feeling rules' were implicit.[2]

It was also evident that feeling rules were not consistent; students were exposed to differing rules ('mixed messages') regarding appropriate feeling and emotional display. For example, in the following focus group discussion, the students contrast the varying responses of qualified midwives following a neonatal death:

Student 1:   The midwife that I was with . . . she never once asked me 'what do you think about it?' and neither did any of the other midwives.

Student 3:   they just let you go early didn't they? . . . Not, 'sit down. Shall we talk about it?'

Student 1:   It was just – 'oh it's sad when it happens, it's part of the job' . . . she said 'you're gonna see it'. But I was lucky because my community midwife was there and she did ask me.

Student 2:   The community midwives do seem to give you that support though, 'cos my community midwife said 'if any time you need me now I'm only a phone call away'. . . .   (FG 3: First-year 18-month students) (Hunter and Deery 2005: 12)

Approaches to managing emotion: Affective neutrality and affective awareness

Data analysis indicated that there were two very different approaches to managing emotion, with differing sets of feeling rules. Put simply, these can be characterised as: affective neutrality (Parsons 1951), that is, the suppression of emotion in order to maintain a 'professional' image; or alternatively affective awareness, aimed at managing emotions via sharing and support. Affective neutrality was more commonly described and observed in the behaviour of hospital midwives, whilst community midwives were more likely to adopt an approach of 'affective awareness'.

These occupational norms regarding emotion are not arbitrary, but interlinked with organisational goals (Sutton 1991). 'Affective neutrality' fits with a 'with institution' ideology (Hunter 2004) aimed at control and reduction of uncertainty. Minimising the emotional content of childbirth is essential in order to rationalise the process and achieve institutional goals. In contrast, a 'with woman' approach focuses on meeting individual women's psychosocial needs; integral to this is acknowledgement of emotional elements of care, as in affective awareness (Hunter 2004). These differing approaches to emotion are discussed in turn.

Affective neutrality

Within the hospital environment, emotion was viewed as an inevitable 'part of the job', that needed to be accepted but suppressed in order for work to continue unimpeded. This attitude was frequently alluded to in the student data. For example, one student wryly commented, after witnessing a traumatic emergency situation:

My mentor said to me 'oh I was going to ask you how you felt but you're back again so you're fine aren't you?' Just because you turned back up again the following morning means it went well yesterday, you're all right!   (FG 2: Final-year 3-year students)

Implicit in this approach is an expectation that emotions will be 'coped with' via individual self-management strategies, as opposed to public acknowledgement and open discussion. Students learnt that they should hide their emotions and deal with them outside of the work setting. In the previous account, the senior midwives constructed the workplace as an emotion-free zone by telling the student to 'go home early'. Whilst on the surface this could be interpreted as a gesture of sympathy, the covert message is that emotion and work are incompatible.

The behaviour and responses of significant others are key factors in the process of learning affective norms. Individuals use 'similarly situated others as a reference group for determining the intensity and quality of contextual emotional experience and expression' (Pogrebin and Poole 1995: 150).

Students appeared to learn very quickly that, in hospital at least, it was not acceptable to reveal that they were upset or angry in front of clients or, perhaps more importantly, in front of more experienced midwives. Being 'emotional' contravened the rational, 'professional' performance that students were aiming to present. The following student describes trying to control her emotions in the presence of a respected senior midwife:

> I didn't want her to see me getting upset again – because I thought she's just going to think I'm some blubbering mass of student who can't get her life together and . . . I've lost any credibility I've had with her already. If I see her again and get upset I'm going to lose even more credibility.   (FG 1: Final-year 18-month students)

Affective neutrality is achieved via individual management of difficulties rather than disclosure. In many occupations feelings are regarded as taboo and hence kept private; workers fear that by revealing their emotional responses, they will be seen as over-emotional and hence inadequate (Smith and Kleinman 1989; Pogrebin and Poole 1995). As in the previous account, becoming upset has implications for occupational credibility.

Affective neutrality may also serve as self-protection for practitioners from uncomfortable feelings; the emotional 'messiness' of work is reduced and rationality, objectivity and efficiency are achieved. However, as will be seen, affective neutrality was not restricted to hospital midwifery. Community-based midwives described situations in which they also adopted an approach of professional detachment.

Affective awareness

At the other end of the spectrum from affective neutrality was affective awareness. Many midwives, particularly those in community-based practice, considered this to be the ideal approach to managing emotions. This affective style has been described by Copp (1998: 304) as 'the professional with a heart'. The focus is on emotional responsiveness and expression, with an emphasis on psychosocial support for both clients and peers. It resonates with a 'with woman' model of practice (Hunter 2004):

> *Midwife 1:* . . . we all talk to each other about things and I find a lot of support comes from colleagues and people.
> *Voices:* It does.
> *Midwife 2:* If somebody's had a bad case . . . I'm thinking of Mary, she was breaking her heart, crying and crying, and we felt so sorry for her . . . she was talking about it and – there but for the grace of god go any of us. [*Voices:* mm] But if you bottle it up, that's where your downfall is. You've got to be able to talk about things.
> (FG 9: F-grade team midwives)

The feeling rules implied in this account clearly differ from affective neutrality. Not only is it acceptable to display emotions, but it is also considered to be of therapeutic value. In line with a contemporary perspective informed by psychoanalysis and counselling theory, the ideal is that of the 'talking cure' – that it is better to express emotions than suppress them (Craib 1994; Fineman 2000). As one midwife commented: 'it's a sort of release valve for you' (FG: nine F-grade team midwives). Empathic support from friends and colleagues provides the means for this 'release'. As Craib (1994) notes, implicit in this approach is the belief that voicing feelings will make them diminish or even disappear, although there is no substantive empirical basis to this belief.

Qualified midwives appeared to divide themselves into 'us and them' groups with regards to expression of emotion: midwives who identified with 'new' midwifery were more likely to present themselves as emotionally expressive, whereas 'old school' midwives were portrayed as 'hard' and out of touch with their feelings. Midwives considered that the rules regarding display of emotion were in the process of changing:

> Midwife 1: midwives have changed haven't they? The sisters were really quite hard . . . You learnt about what to do as a midwife, but you never spoke about your emotions – which they do now – it's much much better . . .
>
> Midwife 3: also maybe being seen as a sign of weakness if you couldn't cope with it [group agreement] whereas now if anybody gets a bad case – they talk for hours and hours about it.
>
> (FG 9: F-grade team midwives)

Lupton (1998) similarly noted a generational difference in attitudes to emotion management. Older participants in her study tended to describe emotions as potentially dangerous and in need of control, whereas younger participants favoured expression of emotions as beneficial for both personal well-being and communication with others.

However, there was also evidence that affective awareness was something of an ideal and that 'talk(ing) for hours and hours' was a rarer occurrence than this account suggests. Community-based midwives frequently found themselves in situations that presented emotional difficulties, leading them to 'retreat' to an affectively neutral approach in order to protect personal boundaries.

Achieving both affective neutrality and affective awareness requires the use of emotion work strategies. 'Impression management' (Goffman 1969) and 'surface acting' (Hochschild 1983) are used to present a facade of coping, whether the end result is a 'cool' or 'warm' persona. Other strategies include withdrawal, 'toughening up' and seeking support.

Emotion work strategies

Impression management: 'an air of calm and reassurance'

In order to present the appropriate calm and objective 'professional performance', felt emotions frequently needed to be controlled and even hidden:

> You daren't show your feelings – you've got to be the smiling supportive practitioner for that woman and her partner. (FG 1: Final-year 18-month students)

Midwives described 'putting on an act' and 'going into role' to achieve this. They displayed emotions that were not actually felt, and described being aware that they were 'faking'. There are similar descriptions of midwifery 'performances' in Ruth Deery's study in Chapter 4.

Acting techniques were used in encounters with both clients and colleagues. Midwives described working at presenting an air of 'calm and reassurance' (FG 10: E- and F-grade hospital midwives) in their encounters with clients, and this was frequently apparent during field-work. For example, I observed one midwife caring for a woman in labour with a twin pregnancy. The fetal heart rate of one of the babies had slowed, a potential indicator of fetal distress. The way in which she let the parents know of her concerns, whilst maintaining an atmos-phere of safety, was evocative of the techniques used by flight atten-dants in Hochschild's (1983: 107) study to create a 'safe homey atmosphere' to avert the fears of anxious passengers:

> A says to the mother 'little righty now – her heartbeat's down to 108 – she might be sleeping but I've asked one of the doctors to come and have a look'. I am struck by the technique that A uses here: she refers to the baby affectionately and as a person, and also as a person who might just be sleeping. She certainly manages to minimise any sense of anxiety, as the parents don't look unduly worried. The atmosphere is calm and relaxed, although I know from discussing the situation with A that she is quite anxious.   (FN 10: E-grade hospital midwife)

I was also struck by the neutral, impassive 'mask' assumed by midwives when dealing with intimate tasks or unpleasant procedures. As Smith and Kleinman (1989: 60) observed in their study of medical students, in such situations practitioners work at transforming the 'inti-mate contact with the body into a mechanical or analytic problem'. One group of student midwives spent some time discussing how they managed the 'problem of the body' (Lawler 1991):

> *Student 1:*   I hadn't realised how personal the whole thing was going to be – and checking the perineum you think 'ooh!' [*group laughter*] that's pretty personal too . . . you're quite embarrassed by it . . .
> *Student 4:*   I think once you get into the role . . . I remember going upstairs with a young girl – she'd had an episiotomy . . . I remem-ber walking up her stairs in the house thinking 'if I was in my own clothes now, not this uniform, I couldn't do it' [*group agreement*]. (FG 4: First-year 3-year students)

This discussion demonstrates the power of performance. By 'getting in the role' and using the relevant artefacts (for example, the uniform), the students transform themselves into neutral professionals, not only in the eyes of clients but also in their own eyes. This also serves to remove the situation from its human (and sexual) context and thus make it more easily manageable.

Although impression management could be used to achieve a facade of professional detachment, it was also used to present a warm and caring image. Midwives described having to consciously 'act the part' of the 'with woman' midwife in situations where they felt emotionally overburdened or 'burnt out':

> *Midwife 1:*   sometimes something awful's happened at home, but you've still got to come in and do this –
>
> *Midwife 2:*   yeah and you've got this face on – that you're going in and [sweetly] 'hello how are you?'
>
> *Midwife 1:*   yeah – I don't really care [group laughter]
>
> *Midwife 3:*   I can't deal with it
>
> *Midwife 4:*   that's right yeah!
>
> *Midwife 3:*   so what! isn't it? I've got problems – I'm not telling you [group laughter]
>
> *Midwife 4:*   that's where midwives are very good actresses
>
> *Midwife 3:*   Oh Christ we're marvellous actresses! We should be having these awards [group laughter] – Oscars for midwives definitely – we are very good actresses! (FG 9: F-grade team midwives) (Hunter and Deery 2005: 13)

Student midwives described using similar impression management strategies. They appeared to experience a 'caring trajectory', as identified by Smith (1992: 112), that is, they became less emotionally involved as their training progressed. Whilst some were concerned by this change, others felt that it reflected a more realistic and sustainable approach:

> *Student 1:*   one thing that I didn't like about myself as I got on, sometimes it just wasn't a magical thing any more you know? [group agreement] Every now and again it was just like something that I did and then I moved on to the next room. When you take a step back and look at yourself sometimes you think 'oh my god!' – this wasn't part of what I thought it would be like – but then other times you do get involved and it is all wonderful again . . .

Student 3: . . . personally I think I couldn't be at work on that emotional kind of extreme all the time – it's just too much [voices in agreement] so I think a lot of the time you are just doing your job but you still *act* in such a way that you know . . . [group agreement] you still give the physical care even if you don't *feel* particularly . . . (FG 2: Final-year 3-year students)

Self-protective barriers: 'switching off' and 'toughening up'

These latter accounts also imply that a sense of detachment may develop. Participants frequently referred to the need to 'switch off' and 'toughen up'. These strategies appeared to be used when midwives felt overwhelmed by circumstances: for example, where midwives were experiencing emotional difficulties in their personal lives; where there were conflicts with colleagues; where workload and time pressures were unmanageable. Relationships with mothers could also present problems if professional and personal boundaries became blurred. This occurred when women had serious social problems for which there was no apparent solution, or when women's expectations of emotional involvement from the midwife were felt to be unrealistic (Hunter 2006). In all these situations, midwives found it difficult to 'act the role', and suppressed their emotions by withdrawing:

Midwife 1:   sometimes you can't afford to be like that [emotionally involved] because there's other issues in your life . . . I sometimes make a conscious decision that today's a turn-off day, because I can't afford to get involved with anything today, because I couldn't cope with any more.   (FG 9: F-grade team midwives)

This account implies a form of emotional withdrawal. There was also evidence of using actual physical distancing, as in the following account where a student described her shock when her mentor carried out a procedure against the client's consent:

It was really horrible – I walked away to the other side of the room and I didn't want any part of it.   (FG 4: First-year 3-year students)

Withdrawal has been noted in other studies of emotion work. Froggatt (1998: 335) found that hospice nurses used 'switching on and off' and 'standing back' as mechanisms to 'metaphorically and mentally distance[d] themselves from the emotional threats engendered by their work'. Withdrawal may also be a strategy for coping with the disparity between occupational ideals and reality. Lipsky (1980) and Copp (1998) argue that disillusioned workers may psychologically withdraw through a process of disengagement with the work, or indeed may totally withdraw by leaving. Although, in the short term, 'switching off' may be an effective method of self-protection, if it is adopted as a long-term strategy, there is a risk of alienation and burnout (Sandall 1997, 1998; Copp 1998; Bakker et al. 2000). There may be clues here to the current problems with retention in midwifery.

'Toughening up' was also used as a means of self-protection. Descriptions of 'becoming hard' appeared frequently in the accounts of students, as in this discussion of peer criticism:

> *Student 1*:   There are little chitchats behind your back 'she does it this way . . . oooo!' . . . so I think you really have to be really strong inside and have to have a very tough exterior, so that when they do say things, it's almost like you've got this protective shield and they bounce off.   (FG 1: Final-year 18-month students)

Community-based midwives providing continuity of care described a similar 'hardening up' process, particularly when they were caring for women with what appeared to be insurmountable social problems:

> You want to sit there and cry with her, 'cause there's not really a lot you can do, except talk to them. You can't say 'well I'll look after the baby for the night'. And yet sometimes you think, if I could do that, she'd be better then tomorrow. You do worry about them. And you have to learn, don't you, to be hard? [group agreement] When I first came out in the community, I was ringing these women up all the time, but I just couldn't do it. (FG 8: F-grade community team midwives)

Self-protective responses such as withdrawal and toughening up are likely to affect the quality of the interaction between worker and client. This may provide a partial explanation for the cool and uncaring behaviours of some midwives noted in various studies (Halldorsdottir and Karlsdottir 1996, Berg et al. 1996; McCrea et al. 1998).

These strategies are also likely to leave midwives feeling isolated, and failing to realise that others may have similar experiences.

Support

Seeking support was a key means of managing emotion. Where midwives were able to provide and receive support this was experienced positively and feelings of isolation were reduced. The cathartic value of talking problems through was frequently alluded to, as was the potential for reframing the situation or seeing it from another perspective. Students frequently made use of their peers for reciprocal emotion management (Lively 2000).

However, support was not always available, accessible or appropriate. Sources of support varied. Hospital midwives were observed to draw on the collegial support provided by their immediate work group, whereas community-based midwives were more likely to turn to clients and specific colleagues. Tensions between midwives could lead to withdrawal of support. In such situations, further emotion work was necessary and midwives described using self-protective strategies and impression management to cope.

It was notable that no midwives mentioned using more formal means of support, such as statutory midwifery supervision. The effectiveness of traditional models of supervision in meeting the support needs of contemporary midwives has been questioned by several authors (Deery and Corby 1996; Kirkham 1999). This is problematic, as unmet support needs have been identified as a key issue in many other contemporary studies of midwifery (Sandall 1997; Kirkham 1999; Kirkham and Stapleton 2000) and a recent study identified lack of support as a significant reason for midwives ceasing to practice (Ball et al. 2002).

Lack of access to effective support can result in long-term distress and emotional damage, as described by this midwife in her account of a harrowing experience that resulted in a maternal death. As a result of the situation, she experienced a 'breakdown', which she attributed to lack of emotional support at the time and her attempts to 'cope' with her feelings alone. She was still clearly affected by the incident several years later:

> *Midwife*: I don't think we had the help and the support we needed . . . and it was just really frightening . . . There was bad communication and not very good support – but I think on the labour ward things happen so fast and terrible things happen and it's just the pace of the place – you just move onto the next one and . . . quite often you don't get the chance to talk things through. I think

> midwives are quite bad at supporting each other . . . nothing was sort of really said – there was just this sort of 'are you all right?' and you know you *had* to say 'yes' – 'right – let's carry on' sort of thing.   (INT: E-grade hospital midwife)

This account clearly illustrates the negative effects of failure to attend to the emotional aspects of work. Support from senior staff was clearly lacking; the emphasis was on suppression of feeling and being seen to 'cope', and the midwife felt unable to challenge this. The account suggests that she was conforming to occupational feeling rules – as she comments, 'you know you *had* to say "yes"'.

The effects of mixed messages

We have seen that there appear to be two different, conflicting approaches to managing emotion in contemporary midwifery, which exist on a continuum from suppression to expression of emotion. Midwives tend towards one approach or the other, but may also change their behaviour along this continuum, often in response to context. Student midwives are well placed to observe these differences, as they work with a variety of senior midwives and clinical mentors. Differences in approach may create difficulties for students, however, as they have to 'suss out' the emotional style of the midwives they are working with and adapt their behaviour.

Lack of a consistent message meant that their peer group became an important reference point. In many focus groups, students were observed to 'test out' their emotional responses and explore the boundaries of acceptability and appropriateness, as in the following discussion. Student 1 has been describing her distress and sense of 'not coping' during an obstetric emergency:

> *Billie*:   what was it you felt you couldn't cope with?
> *Student 1*:   I think – of not crying – of not being in control of the situation – because I could see her husband and he was so distraught and upset and . . . I just thought that I would be absolutely useless because I'd be crying with him and I thought hmmmm. . . .
> *Student 2*:   but that's acceptable
> *Student 3*:   yeah – you are of use by comforting him – that is one of the hardest jobs I think isn't it?

Student 2:   and if you cry with him that's fine
Student 3:   yeah
Student 1:   [doubtfully] is it acceptable?
Student 4:   yeah, I think it is actually.   (FG 1: Final-year 18-month students)

Contradictory rules regarding emotional display are evident in this discussion. Student 1 appeared to have accepted the rule regarding the need for emotional control and was self-critical of the difficulties she experienced in achieving this. However, other students challenged this and introduced an opposing feeling rule: that crying is not only 'fine' but also an effective means of client support.

There were similar accounts in other focus group discussions, and it was evident that students were frequently confused about how best to manage emotions. Although many held an ideal of an emotionally aware style of practice, they frequently conformed to the dominant approach of affective neutrality. One student described an intimate and highly emotional situation in which she had spent many hours caring for a woman who had given birth to a baby with Down's Syndrome. She later explained that, although she wished to visit the woman and baby at home, she considered that this would be unacceptable within the cultural norms of midwifery:

Student 1:   They're always on my mind and I'm not living far away from them and yet I know it's not appropriate to knock at the door . . . and yet I want to know . . .
Billie: Why do you feel it's not appropriate?
Student 1:   Am I overstepping the mark? Am I becoming too involved? [*group agreement*] Is it professional?   (FG 2: Final-year 3-year students)

The student's behaviour was clearly determined with reference to occupational norms: her personal desire for continued client contact was suppressed in accordance with the perceived feeling rules regarding maintenance of 'professional' boundaries and reduction of personal involvement.

Learning how best to manage emotions was thus a trial and error process, with novice midwives learning informally by picking up 'clues' from senior midwives and peers. Further research could usefully explore how this results in the differing emotional 'styles' observed in qualified midwives.

Conclusion

The findings of this study suggest that a continuum of approaches to emotion management exist within contemporary UK midwifery. The ideal held by many midwives was to work in an affectively aware manner. However, such an approach was often unsustainable and, as a result, midwives resorted to affective neutrality. This may explain the findings of McCrea et al. (1998), who observed labour ward midwives exhibiting styles which they categorised as the 'cold professional', the 'warm professional' and the 'disorganised carer'. However, rather than these styles being fixed characteristics of each midwife, as McCrea et al. (1998) suggest, they are more likely to be contextually located responses to the demands of the work, and midwives may oscillate between approaches. This is experienced by novices as 'mixed messages', which may prove challenging during the socialisation process.[3]

How women and their families experience midwives' differing approaches to emotion management was not explored within this research. Evidence from other studies suggests that women are very much aware of the differing 'styles' of their midwives (Halldorsdottir and Karlsdottir 1996; Berg et al. 1996; McCrea et al. 1998) and that the quality of their childbirth experience is inevitably affected by this. The chapters in this book by Chris McCourt and Trudy Stevens, and Nadine Edwards (Chapters 1 and 2) also provide moving accounts of women's emotional experiences. It is very likely to be the case that women, as well as novice midwives, will experience 'mixed messages'.

So how can midwives work in ways that are emotionally supportive to women and also ensure that they attend carefully to their own emotional needs? Surely the two are not mutually exclusive? A common phrase used by midwives was the need to 'get the balance right' in relation to emotion management, so that both work and personal lives were kept in harmony, and stress and burnout were avoided. It is very important that we develop our understanding of how midwives can best achieve (and sustain) this, in order to nurture the emotional well-being of midwives and hence enhance the quality of care given to women and their families. There are some clues provided by the studies of caseload midwifery (Stevens and McCourt 2002; Chris McCourt and Trudy Stevens, Chapter 1) and birth centre care (Walsh 2007), which suggest that reciprocal relationships are of key importance.

We also need to explore how to support the development of midwives' emotion work skills and emotional awareness. Other authors have suggested that forum theatre (see Kirsten Baker's chapter in this book) and clinical supervision (Deery and Corby 1996) may provide effective tools for assisting this development. Further research is urgently needed to investigate how midwives can best be supported to become skilled 'emotion workers'.

Reflective questions

1 Have you seen midwives using 'affectively neutral' and 'affectively aware' approaches? What impact do you think these approaches have on the experiences of (a) mothers and (b) colleagues?

2 Have you experienced 'mixed messages' regarding emotion management? If so, has this created difficulties for you?

3 What would help you in developing your skills in managing emotion?

Notes

1 In the data extracts, FG denotes a focus group; FN denotes field notes and INT denotes an interview. All extracts are anonymised.
2 'Feeling rules' are social norms regarding what should be felt and what should be displayed in differing social contexts. For further discussion, see the introduction to this book.
3 However, one potential benefit is that 'mixed messages' may provide novices with insights into a range of approaches, so that they are able to evaluate each and find their own 'emotional style'.

References

Bakker, A. B., Schaufeli, W. B., Sixma, H. J., Bosveld, W. and van Dierendonck, D. (2000) Patient demands, lack of reciprocity, and burnout: a five-year longitudinal study among general practitioners, *Journal of Organizational Behavior*, 21: 425–41.

Ball, L., Curtis, P. and Kirkham, M. (2002) *Why Do Midwives Leave?* Women's Informed Childbearing and Health Research Group, University of Sheffield.

Berg, M., Lundgren, I., Hermansson, E. and Wahlberg, V. (1996) Women's experience of the encounter with the midwife during childbirth, *Midwifery*, 12: 11–15.

Bolton, S. C. (2000) Who cares? Offering emotion work as a 'gift' in the nursing labour process, *Journal of Advanced Nursing*, 32(3): 580–6.

Bosk, C. L. (1979) *Forgive and Remember: Managing Medical Failure* (Chicago: University of Chicago Press).

Copp, M. (1998) When emotion work is doomed to fail: Ideological and structural constraints of emotion management, *Symbolic Interaction*, 21(3): 299–328.

Craib, I. (1994) *The Importance of Disappointment* (London: Routledge).

Deery, R. and Corby, D. (1996) A case for clinical supervision in midwifery. In: M. Kirkham (ed.), *Supervision of Midwives* (Hale, Cheshire: Books for Midwives Press), pp. 203–12.

Fineman, S., ed. (2000) *Emotion in Organizations*, 2nd edn (London: Sage).

Froggatt, K. (1998) The place of metaphor and language in exploring nurses' emotional work, *Journal of Advanced Nursing*, 28(2): 332–8.

Goffman, E. (1969) *The Presentation of Self in Everyday Life* (London: Allen Lane, Penguin Press).

Halldorsdottir, S. and Karlsdottir, S. I. (1996) Journeying through labour and delivery: perceptions of women who have given birth, *Midwifery*, 12: 48–61.

Hochschild, A. R. (1983) *The Managed Heart: Commercialization of Human Feeling* (Berkeley, CA: University of California Press).

Hunter, B. (2002) Emotion work in midwifery. Unpublished PhD thesis, University of Wales Swansea.

Hunter, B. (2004) Conflicting ideologies as a source of emotion work in midwifery, *Midwifery*, 20: 261–72.

Hunter, B. (2005) Emotion work and boundary maintenance in hospital-based midwifery, *Midwifery*, 21: 253–66.

Hunter, B. (2006) The importance of reciprocity in relationships between community-based midwives and mothers, *Midwifery*, 22(4), 308–22.

Hunter, B. and Deery, R. (2005) Building our knowledge about emotion work in midwifery: combining and comparing findings from two different research studies, *Evidence Based Midwifery*, 3(1): 10–15.

Kirkham, M. (1999) The culture of midwifery in the National Health Service in England, *Journal of Advanced Nursing*, 30(3): 732–9.

Kirkham, M. and Stapleton, H. (2000) Midwives' support needs as childbirth changes, *Journal of Advanced Nursing*, 32(2): 465–72.

Lawler, J. (1991) *Behind the Screens: Nursing, Somology and the Problem of the Body* (Edinburgh: Churchill Livingstone).

Lipsky, M. (1980) *Street-Level Bureaucracy: Dilemmas of the Individual in Public Services* (New York: Russell Sage Foundation).

Lively, K. J. (2000) Reciprocal emotion management: working together to maintain stratification in private law firms, *Work and Occupations*, 27(1): 32–63.

Lupton, D. (1998) *The Emotional Self* (London: Sage).

McCrea, H., Wright, M. and Murphy-Black, T. (1998) Differences in midwives' approaches to pain relief in labour, *Midwifery*, 14: 174–80.

Parsons, T. (1951) *The Social System* (New York: Free Press).

Pogrebin, M. R. and Poole, E. D. (1995) Emotion management: a study of police response to tragic events, *Social Perspectives on Emotion*, 3: 149–68.

Sandall, J. (1997) Midwives' burnout and continuity of care, *British Journal of Midwifery*, 5(2): 106–11.

Sandall, J. (1998) Midwifery work, family life and wellbeing: a study of occupational change. Unpublished PhD thesis, University of Surrey, Guildford.

Smith, A.C. and Kleinman, S. (1989) Managing emotions in medical school: students' contacts with the living and the dead, *Social Psychology Quarterly*, 52(1): 56–69.

Smith, P. (1992) *The Emotional Labour of Nursing* (Basingstoke: Palgrave Macmillan).

Stevens, T. and McCourt, C. (2002) One-to-one midwifery practice, part 3: Meaning for midwives, *British Journal of Midwifery*, 10(2): 111–15.

Sutton, R. I. (1991) Maintaining norms about expressed emotions: the case of the bill collectors, *Administrative Science Quarterly*, 36: 245–68.

Walsh, D. (2007) *Improving Maternity Services: Small is Beautiful – Lessons from a Birth Centre* (Oxford: Radcliffe Publishing).

11

Inner Knowing and Emotions in the Midwife–Woman Relationship

Ólöf Ásta Ólafsdóttir

Introduction

This chapter will explore how the 'inner knowing' of midwives develops though their relationships with women, as illustrated in their birth stories which embrace the emotional experiences of midwifery practice. 'Inner knowing' is also known as 'intuitive knowledge'. I will begin by briefly describing the research journey of my PhD study (Ólafsdóttir 2006), on which this chapter is based, before discussing the findings related to different kinds of 'inner knowing' in midwifery.

The study was conducted in Iceland, one of the Nordic countries where around 300,000 people live and there are about 4500 births per year (Statistics Iceland 2008). It is a very small society in a country of 103,000 km^2, the most sparsely populated country in Europe with 63 per cent wasteland and people living around the coastal belt in urban centres (Halldórsson 2003). About 3000 of these births take place in the central university hospital in the capital town of Reykjavik, where most of the population live. The remainder take place out in the countryside, where midwives work at community health centres and/or small hospitals. In many places women have to travel away from home for between 1 and 3 hours to give birth. The number of births per place of birth in rural and remote areas varies from a total of 15 to 400 per year (Geirsson et al. 2006). Thus, due to centralisation of maternity services, places of birth differ regarding size and busyness and also in opportunities to provide continuity of care. This affects the midwife's potential for knowing and being with the woman and her family around childbirth.

Narrative analysis was used to identify the plot (Polkinghorne 1995) of midwives' birth stories. When the many threads of the midwives' stories were drawn together, the unifying thematic plots of 'being with' woman and 'safety' were identified as linking and directing the core narrative of midwifery in Iceland. This core narrative refers to how the act of 'being with' or 'sitting over' (in Icelandic *yfirseta*) the woman during birth is fundamental to learning and developing midwifery skills. In particular, it facilitates making connections with the woman and the birth itself, so that midwives learn to trust and listen to their inner voice and develop different types of 'inner knowing'. These are in balance with other types of knowledge systems in midwifery practice, such as theoretical knowledge derived from obstetrics and biomedicine. 'Inner knowing' is the term I use for different types of intuitive knowledge, which were inextricably linked to midwives' relationships with women, particularly the emotional and spiritual connections. As one midwife told me: 'you are not able to learn it elsewhere. You are just able to learn it there, with the woman'.

The aims and process of the study

The aim of this research was to explore storytelling about Icelandic midwives' working lives, in the period from the mid-twentieth century to the present time. It was based on the belief that birth stories of midwives are a mine full of their knowledge, which could be uncovered by ethnographic narrative methods. Interviews were conducted with 20 midwives with different backgrounds (in relation to education, length of clinical experience and birth setting) from all over the country, in order to collect birth stories that represented the social and cultural world of childbirth and midwifery. Furthermore, one focus group interview with six midwives was conducted and field notes were made. Theory was to arise inductively from the midwives' own telling, in order to identify their authentic voice of midwifery ideology and knowledge. The midwives' storytelling reinforced different aspects of their own values (Kirkham 1997) and it was challenging to put my own previous ideas aside to wait for and look at what ideas emerged from the midwives' stories.

Early on, while narrowing down the focus of study, the different aspects of the concept of inner knowing began to emerge. In the first interviews, older midwives who had worked alone out in the countryside for decades told stories of feeling that 'they were not alone' and of having 'the sixth sense' when they attended births. These stories were unprompted and surprised me and made me interested in going on to explore this spiritual side of midwifery.

You are not alone, for example when you are breaking down because you are very tired and maybe anxious, then you go aside and talk to someone [and you receive some energy to go on]. There is someone who has been a guide. I do not believe in psychic things but I feel that I have had guidance from someone we can call god . . . it is like the sixth sense is behind which you cannot identify.   (Midwife, Elsa, with 50 years' experience)

From then on, I asked all the midwives if they had had the same experience and explored with them what the meaning of this could be. All the midwives who had worked in the countryside had this kind of experience, but were not sure what it was and related this to their inner voice or inner knowing. For example, one midwife said that, as she had been 'lucky', she therefore assumed she had help from another world and that she was not the only midwife who felt this. The midwives also talked about being in touch with God or someone who gave strength or helped them to go on. They felt that this enabled them to be rational and make the right clinical decisions. All these experiences were also related to different aspects of their relationships with the woman, especially when these were reciprocal and empowering.

As a result of this unexpected finding, the interviews were developed to explore the midwives' relationship with the woman at birth, focusing on their inner knowing or intuition and how this linked to experience and/or spirituality. In particular, I wanted to explore what this kind of midwifery knowledge consists of and how it develops. Three different types of inner knowing were identified, and these will be presented and discussed, using midwives' birth stories. Before exploring the concept of inner knowing further, I will briefly discuss the importance for the midwives of forming close connections with women.

Close connections and emotional experiences

Midwifery is to be there when you are needed and help the parents at this wonderful moment in their life. I think that is the core . . . I feel I am a friend, as if I am one of the family, when I am with them [the women]. Like a family friend even though you are not related or that you don't know them a lot. It is just that you are so close, yes in close connection and cooperation and it is touching and there are strong emotions and I experience them with them.   (Midwife, Rosa, with 25 years' experience)

From the perspective of this narrative from one of the country midwives, effective midwifery care relies on strong emotions arising from close connections with the woman and her family. Meaningful relationships between midwives and mothers are one of the elements identified as central to contemporary paradigms of midwifery practice (Siddiqui 1999, 2005; Kirkham 2000; Page 2004; Pairman 2006). A growing body of knowledge shows that midwives' relationships with women, particularly the emotional support offered, are important in ensuring positive experiences which will have an effect on people for a long time (Mander 2001; Sauls 2002; Deery and Kirkham 2006; Hodnett 2006a, 2006b; Hodnett et al. 2006).

These relationships inevitably generate emotions. As discussed by other authors in this book, dealing with emotions is an important and demanding component of working with people, entailing management of feelings and expression of emotion (Hunter 2001, 2004). In this study, the connections and the emotions they generated were seen as integral to the development of ways of knowing in midwifery practice. As the midwife above says: midwifery is the midwife and woman 'in close connection and cooperation and it is touching and there are strong emotions and I experience them with them'.

Defining inner knowing and spirituality

Defining inner knowing of midwives is difficult and by attempting to do so we may be in danger of restricting the full and complex meaning, particularly how it may relate to clinical skills. The same can be said about attempts to define spirituality. Definitions of spirituality are often linked to human relationships and are seen as part of being able to give and receive love and give practical care (Hall 2001; Hall and Taylor 2004). There is evidence in the literature that midwives allude to the challenges of birth and providing sensitive care to women in ways that appear spiritual (Leap 2000; Page 2004; Page and McCandlish 2006). By working as a 'skilled companion' (Page 1993: 4), the midwife, through her connective ways of knowing, combines clinical skills and scientific knowledge with an inner sensitivity to this significant event as a new circle of life begins.

Hall (2001) has pointed out how the spiritual aspects of midwifery have received little attention in midwifery discourse, education and research. She identified multifactorial elements of spirituality from reviewing health care literature. These included: transcendence, search for meaning and purpose, connecting, relational aspects, self-awareness, hope and faith. Applying these to childbirth and the midwife–woman relationship, Hall (2001) suggested that human relationship is needed by the spirit and that spirituality is demonstrated through actions to others.

Inner knowing is also problematic to define. It was discussed and articulated in various ways by the Icelandic midwives in this study, but when the literature was searched to find similarities, little previous research was found. The exception was the study by Davis-Floyd and Davis (1997) about intuition as authoritative knowledge, based on interviews with 22 home birth midwives in the USA. Those midwives were found to use a type of care based on intuition, which seemed to involve body and the spirit but not necessarily the rational mind. Intuition emerged 'out of their own inner connectedness to the deepest bodily and spiritual aspects of their being as well as out of their physical and psychic connections to the mother and the child' (Davis-Floyd and Davis 1997: 339). This description fits well with the narratives of inner ways of knowing of Icelandic midwives, who described it as an ongoing process of 'this sense that comes' from within the self:

> I think all midwives learn from themselves. We learn and find out what there is inside us. It is a combination of skills and intuition and being able to unite it. It is this sense that comes when you know if everything is normal or not.   (Midwife, Bella, with 6 years' experience)

Thus inner knowing in relation to the emotional and spiritual aspects of childbirth is incorporated as a dimension of midwifery practice but in a silent way, as a 'tacit' knowledge. This tacit knowledge has been in part uncovered and described in the midwifery narratives of this study.

As described earlier, midwives who worked in the countryside described their feeling of 'not being alone' at a birth; rather there was someone giving them inner strength. Other midwives identified with this feeling. Although this was not an experience of all participants, many described this, even if they did not have long practice experience or only had working experience on a busy hospital labour ward:

> I am definitely a little bit crazy, I feel that someone is with me, I have always had this feeling that someone good is with me. I only have to learn to trust this . . . [gives an example about when she had premonition of shoulder dystocia, and should have called earlier for assistance, for someone to be with her.]   (Midwife, Sigrid, with 6 years' experience)

This attention to inner knowing and intuition is in contrast to the claim by Hall and Taylor (2004) that nowadays UK midwifery students are losing intuitive skills very early on, or even missing the chance to develop them. They attribute this to the decrease in attendance at physiological births.

As in Sigrid's narrative above, some midwives used the term 'crazy' about their experiences of inner knowing, which suggests that this kind of knowing is not valued by others or considered to be authoritative knowledge in midwifery practice. However, despite this, they appeared to value it themselves and did not talk about it as being mystical but rather described it in a very down-to-earth way, part of being human. For example, discussing an inner voice of spirituality and close connection, Eva defined inner knowing as:

> it is something of being human everywhere. I think it is the same thing, what parents have to develop as human beings, which you develop in challenging situations . . . The midwife also has this great human closeness. She is in a very close connection with her client, both physically and spiritually. Maybe it becomes spiritual because you are allowed to touch the person physically, maybe there is some fusion there, because there are not any brick walls, that prohibit you to touch and when this happens one is moved before the other. (Midwife, Eva, with 28 years' experience)

A common thread between the midwives' stories was how inner knowing is developed by being present with the woman. It is through connection with her that they find it inside themselves and learn to listen to it. Furthermore they described how this knowledge is a combination of skills and knowledge, and of gathering different information from their unconscious mind. They felt that this knowing helps them to be confident in their work, and to become empowered to go on and ensure the safety of the mother and the baby.

Types and use of inner knowing

As mentioned before, three types of inner knowing were identified from the midwives' stories: intuition based on practice experience, intuition based on spiritual awareness and intuition based on connective knowing with the woman. These are illustrated in the form of a model (Figure 11.1), which shows the overlapping and integration of different types of inner knowing.

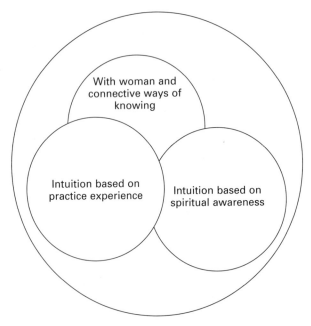

Figure 11.1   Inner knowing in midwifery in balance with other knowledge systems

The first type (intuition based on practice experience) is described in the nursing literature as pattern recognition that occurs in response to experience and expert knowledge in practice (Benner 1984; Dreyfus and Dreyfus 1996). This is a trigger for nursing action and/or reflection and has a direct bearing on interventions in practice (King and Appleton 1997). This kind of knowledge becomes internalised and the practitioner cannot always explain these intuitive judgements and decisions.

The second type (intuition based on spiritual awareness) is more mystical or supernatural and is even more difficult to acknowledge or understand. It gets very little attention in discussions or research into midwifery knowledge. This kind of evidence sits firmly outside the realms of normal science and so-called rational thinking (Wickham 2004: 165).

The third type ('with woman' and connective ways of knowing) reflects the descriptions of intuition as inner connectedness between the midwife and the woman (Davis-Floyd and Davis 1997). Descriptions of this type of knowing suggested that it contained overlapping elements of Types 1 and 2. This type of knowing was enhanced by the connection between the midwife and woman. It develops on different levels in an integrated way and was considered to be in balance with other kind of knowledge systems.

The following narratives that speak for themselves have been chosen to represent the different types of inner knowing.

1. Intuition based on practice experience

This must be the experience. . . . It could be the subconscious mind that gathers information, that comes up when you need it, and out in the country you are always checking if everything is fine, and then you get this feeling . . . I do not know why, just this feeling inside you, there was this woman giving birth with her second baby, and everything goes well, the heartbeat and such, and the woman is fine. Her belly is different, but she did not have the contractions ring, you know, as should be if you suspect danger of a uterus rupture, but this not as it should be. She had CTG and the strip was fine, and she did not complain very much, but there was something. It is maybe foolish to say this but it was strange to examine her, okay I am there for the next hours [continues to describe how she is constantly checking, comparing different symptoms to the situation]. Another midwife came on shift and I tell her, that I do not know, but that I am not satisfied with this, there is something there, when you palpate her belly, something does not fit, that I have been on my toes for two hours. I said: 'go on being on your toes'. She had a caesarean an hour later, the heartbeat changed suddenly and the contractions ring appeared and she was just in surgery when the uterus started to rupture. I called a doctor, because I just had to tell him that I was not satisfied, and he understood what I meant but did not see anything either. This is possibly the strangest thing I have experienced. I could not put my finger on it, but I listened to this feeling because it was so strong.   (Midwife, Monica, with 36 years' experience)

This appears to describe intuitive knowledge, defined as 'subjective, contextualized and transcended through new experiences' (Johns 2000: 43) which is based on pattern recognition by the expert practitioner. This type of knowing also links to the spiritual kind.

2.   *Intuition based on spiritual awareness*

> This is something else [than practice experience] because I felt this right after graduation, then I had this sense, and it could not be experience, and I thought it might be me not being confident, but this goes on . . . and this is not less or more, if you can talk about this in magnitudes. It just pops up once in a while: 'this should not be like this', or 'this is not going to go well'. It is something, I do not know what it is, and you have this not such a good feeling. First you were insecure and you often thought, is this just nonsense? – But now I have more experience and I have the confidence. The walk to the phone [to call for advice] used to be shorter [laughs]. I know that intuition is telling me the right thing. I think it grows and with experience you begin to believe in it, when you get more confident you learn to believe that this is *a sense* instead of *'non-sense'*. It is not the same thing; it is like the intuition grows with the experience but not that it necessarily is dependent on it.   (Midwife, Kristine, with 2 years' experience)

Thus even relatively newly qualified midwives draw on intuition that seems to be derived from 'somewhere else', not necessarily experience.

3.   *'With-woman' and connective ways of knowing*

Below is a story that illustrates the connective ways of knowing of midwife Eva, her sensitive care when she uses her inner knowing based on her practice experience, spiritual awareness and professional knowledge, balancing her knowledge and skills from different knowledge systems. She connects with the woman, assesses the whole situation and decides to be always at this woman's side. In good co-operation with the doctor she 'breaks the rules' by using her connective knowing that emphasises not autonomy and independence of judgement but joining of minds (Belenky et al. 1997). This emotionally charged story is about how the mother feels that the midwife must be as hungry as she is after the birth, both being in primal need of getting back the energy they spent together, as one person. The midwife may have managed her emotions in a positive way by leaving the room to 'have a cry'.

> This woman was in death's anguish and was not able to communicate with words. She had lost a lot; there had been sickness and death

around her. She had also had a premature baby before and this one was just under 36 weeks. I am not quite sure but I think she did not have any baby alive. And she just was not there, and I just allowed her – and decided always to be by her side. The heartbeat went down and the baby was delivered by vacuum extraction. I got this strong feeling that she just had to have her baby in her arms. There was a shift change but I did not go home. The sugar level went down and I did what was necessary there with the woman, provided intensive care for the baby in her arms and helped her with breastfeeding. When this story took place, this baby would have gone to the neonatal intensive care, now this has changed and this kind of care, keeping the woman and baby together, is a part of the routine care at the labour ward. – Because of the rules I was so afraid that she would not be allowed to have her baby with her to the postnatal and I had to leave the room to have a cry about that – After some time she suddenly took a deep breath and looked at me and said: 'Are you, not getting hungry? At this moment we were one, she knew it and I knew it. I knew I was doing the right thing. She went to the postnatal ward with her chubby baby, breastfeeding, and she milked a lot even though she was under stress. In all this I worked very well with the resident paediatrician, he understood very well what I was doing, and I think warmly of him.   (Midwife, Eva, with 28 years' experience)

Linking emotional experiences and development of inner knowing

The midwives' stories suggested that development of inner knowing was often related to emotional situations. These could be positive or negative situations, such as when celebrating beautiful births or grieving the death of a newborn. These emotions could support or restrict development of inner knowing depending on the context.

Negative situations included midwives' relationships with their women, which were not always beneficial and could be emotionally difficult, creating emotion work. Stories were also told about when things went wrong, about events that perhaps help to develop emotional awareness and ways to manage emotions, stories which the midwife 'would like to be without':

Of course it sits in your mind . . . a story you would like to be without. I got a very difficult shoulder dystocia and I just could not get the baby out, it was so difficult – It was difficult and it still is. It was the doctor who got the baby. He, this wonderful boy was harmed and lived only for a few months and it was because of the birth, but the heartbeat was fine. This is something you don't want to happen. I would have liked to be without this story.   (Midwife, Rosa, with 25 years' experience)

The different types of inner knowing such as the spiritual are likely to grow during this kind of experience, that is, when the midwife encounters complex situations around childbirth, and has to deal with emergencies to save life. When Rebecca told a story about how she assessed a woman who had an impending uterine rupture and had to fight to get her an emergency Caesarean, she said:

I think I have someone, without doubt, someone who is fond of me and goes behind me, even though I have not been looking for this [because she is not psychic]. It just is there, when you need it. (Midwife, Rebecca, with 45 years' experience)

Although the midwives in this study experienced strong emotions and spiritual relationships as rewarding and even empowering, just like midwives in the UK they also experience stress and burnout. Birth stories included negative experiences of the working environment which made the midwives feel disempowered. As one midwife with 18 years' practice experience, 11 of which were on the busy labour ward at the university hospital, described:

I fight the battle between these feelings of liking my profession, which today gives me pain, rather than fulfilment, and the feelings of not being able to stay on the job. When I go home, there are very few shifts when I think: today I have been a midwife, working with my woman, helping her to take on this strange journey of pain that the birth is, helping her to be a strong woman. There are constant examples of when I am performing tasks that are far too many for one person. I even have two women at the same time, where one is not as far along as the other woman who a year ago required a continuous 'sitting over' but today she cannot be assured that she is going to have it.   (field notes, a midwife's diary in May 2004)

Negative emotions and experiences such as those in the narrative above affect the development of inner knowing. The presence of the midwife 'being with woman' was in this study identified as crucial for preserving and developing inner knowing. This midwife was concerned because her woman could not be reassured of having a midwife at her side during birth. Her work 'gives her pain', which is a source for emotion work (Hunter 2004, 2005). Just as UK studies have shown, these kinds of working patterns and staff shortages result in exhaustion and burnout as well as the need for professional support (Kirkham and Stapleton, 2000; Deery 2005; Deery and Kirkham 2006). This occurs particularly in fragmented centralised maternity services where the workload has been increasing and midwives have to base their work on conflicting models of care (Hunter 2004; Deery 2005; Ólafsdóttir 2006).

Thus the context in which care is given may enhance inner knowing or reduce opportunities for its development. Calm surroundings and opportunities for the woman to have the midwife at her side appear to be highly important not just for the woman but also for the midwife, in order for her to preserve and hold on to midwifery skills and ways of knowing. Midwives often made comments similar to those of Monika, when she says that 'there has to be certain calm' in order for inner knowing to develop:

> I get this feeling, but there has to be certain calm, I need to be in a peaceful mind, I am not running – when I get this feeling or when instinct works with me. Then I would be doing something for the woman in calm surroundings. It is not only when I have to be on the toes, or when I sense problems coming up. I can just as well get this feeling when everything is normal. This natural event is happening and you are doing your best, guiding the parents. *I call this connection* . . ., it is not exactly that, it is in the unconscious mind.   (Midwife, Monika, with 36 years' experience)

Many authors would agree that calm is important for successful birth (see Berg et al. 1996; Halldórsdóttir and Karlsdóttir 1996; Fleming 1998; Kirkham 2000; Page 2000). Leap and Edwards (2006) also claim that the relationship between women and their known midwife is helpful to create this calm, and will decrease the influences of the technocratic birth culture. As Monika warns us, if the midwife is 'running' and not 'with woman', she can't hear her inner voice, or attend to her midwifery skills and experience and must therefore increasingly rely on textbook knowledge and accumulated experience from routine medicalised practice. Similarly, the home birth midwives in America interviewed by Davis-Floyd and Davis (1997) claimed that there were degrees or levels of connections that they could maintain with the mother and the child. Thus tranquillity can be seen as crucial for professional development, for carers to be aware of their own flow of thoughts, feelings and emotions.

Birth stories to learn from – development of emotional awareness

Underlying the use of a narrative research approach is the belief that people make sense of their world most effectively by telling stories (Bailey and Tilley 2002). Stories become stand-ins for lived experience. Drawing on the work of Benner (1984), I also suggest that they enable us to identify midwifery knowledge, and provide exemplars to learn from or to inform developments of midwifery practice, education and research. Midwives gain skills through effective storytelling (Kirkham 1997), for example, by facilitating discussion and analysis of the professional challenges that relate to emotional awareness and work in midwifery and childbirth care.

In this chapter, relevant narratives and birth stories have been used to highlight the three different types of inner knowing. They include events and views that incorporate the emotion work involved in being a midwife, particularly in relationships with women. I suggest that they can be used to learn from in order to develop emotional and spiritual awareness. When you read or hear them you can draw from them, learn about inner knowing as a part of the emotional nature of midwifery practice and link this to other stories happening in your own environment or in different places of birth and other countries.

Cultural context and inner knowing

This study focuses only on the experiences and birth stories of Icelandic midwives, and it is not possible to know whether their experiences are unique or shared by midwives in other cultures. Nordic mythology, the magic of nature, superstition and beliefs in fate and predestination are all embedded in Icelandic culture. *Huldufólk, or 'hidden* people', are still to be found. This is not only in living memory as a strong image of the nation (Harding and Bindloss 2004), handed down from generation to generation and in folktales (Árnason 1961; Jónasson, 1961); *huldufólk* also appear regularly in the media, such as when they disturb builders of houses. Many folktales also deal with midwives who helped and attended births of the hidden people. If midwives were thought to be incredibly lucky in their work, it was considered to be a sign of something supernatural or that they got help from the hidden people or the fairies. They were paid with the pledge that the midwives and their families would have a happy life and often they also gave presents – beautiful clothes made of silk or pieces of silver (Sigurðardóttir 1984). Possibly these kinds of national and cultural traits could, in part, account for midwives' connections with their inner knowing.

In their accounts the midwives drew attention to the fact that they were not psychic, but rather that they were sensitive to people and their surroundings. They discussed believing in a higher power like God, but this was not necessarily based on religious belief. It is notable that anthropological studies also describe this 'matter of fact' type of knowing, and the value that it is accorded in indigenous societies. For example, in the far reaches of the tropical rainforest in Malaysia, midwife De Ode also found strength in having someone behind:

> We call the spirit Raib and it is like the wind, it cannot be seen, but we know that it is good and will help us when we need it. The delivery of a child is easy when the spirit is around.   (De Ode, quoted by Vincent-Priya 1991: 151)

It is interesting to wonder whether Icelandic midwives have or need a sense of 'someone behind' because of the great responsibilities and challenges that are inherent in midwifery work. They also might need to draw on this type of knowledge within a culture of medically dominated practice because they lack confidence in their own authentic professional knowledge. However, it could be the other way around: that is, that they are confident and empowered because they have this higher power, a form of spiritual guidance which is with them as part of their inner, hidden legitimate knowing in their culture of midwifery practice. By personal experience midwives who have this kind of authoritative inner knowing on which their actions are based (Jordan 1997) are often highly respected by their colleague midwives and doctors in practice.

Conclusions

Inner knowing in midwifery practice is a silent knowledge that is in part uncovered in the midwifery narrative presented in this chapter. The different types of inner knowing interplay with different knowledge systems in the maternity services, from positivist scientific knowledge to spiritual guidance. Connective knowing, derived from the midwife's relationship with the woman and the woman's own power and knowledge about her birth, has the potential to increase midwifery knowledge and skills.

It is clear that my study raises lots of questions that require more investigation. Through fascinating storytelling, the wholeness of the experience of inner knowing of Icelandic midwives appears not so much in words as in atmosphere. For example, one of the home birth midwives, Linda, described how she can sense if the baby has already been born when she arrives, as the home changes. Birth stories are often told in a language that includes the spiritual experience of life, of the spirit or soul being born, wherever the birth takes place.

It is suggested that the midwife–woman relationship and the related emotional experiences (whether they are positive or negative), may affect the development of midwifery skills and the inner knowing of midwives. It is paramount that we should go on exploring and developing concepts that refer to the different kind of inner knowing, emotional and spiritual experiences in midwifery practice. More in-depth research is needed to explore how the forming of relationships between the midwife and the woman affects development of midwifery skills and knowledge in general, as well as how this affects the experiences of women and their families in different cultures and places of birth.

Reflective questions

1   This chapter explores what Icelandic midwives mean by 'inner knowing'. What do you think midwives in the country where you practise would understand by this term?

2   Do you think that the different kinds of 'inner knowing' that have been outlined in this chapter are something that midwives should, and could, develop?

3   Can you tell a story from your own practice that you have learned from, where the relationship with the woman and her family helped you to develop your emotional or spiritual awareness?

References

Árnason, J. (1961/1862) *Íslenskar thjódsögur og aefintýri*, vol. I [Icelandic folklore and folktales], 2nd edn (Reykjavík: Bókaútgáfan Thjódsaga).

Bailey, P. H. and Tilley, S. (2002) Storytelling and the interpretation of meaning in qualitative research, *Journal of Advanced Nursing*, 38(6): 574–83.

Belenky, M. F., Clinchy, B. M., Goldberger, N. R. and Tarule, J. M. (1997) *Women's Ways of Knowing: The Development of Self, Voice, and Mind*, 10th anniversary edn (New York: Basic Books).

Benner, P. E. (1984) *From Novice to Expert: Excellence and Power in Clinical Nursing Practice* (Menlo Park, CA: Addison-Wesley, Nursing Division).

Berg, M., Lundgren, I., Hermansson, E. and Wahlberg, V. (1996) Women's experience of the encounter with the midwife during childbirth, *Midwifery*, 12(1): 11–15.

Davis-Floyd, R. and Davis, E. (1997) Intuition as authoritative knowledge in midwifery and home birth. In: R. Davis-Floyd and C. F. Sargent (eds), *Childbirth and Authoritative Knowledge: Cross-cultural Perspectives* (Berkeley, CA: University of California Press).

Deery, R. (2005) An action-research study exploring midwives' support needs and the effect of group clinical supervision, *Midwifery*, 21(2): 161–76.

Deery, R. and Kirkham, M. (2006) Supporting midwives to support women. In: L. A. Page and R. McCandlish (eds), *The New Midwifery: Science and Sensitivity in Practice*, 2nd edn (Edinburgh: Churchill Livingstone).

Dreyfus, H. L. and Dreyfus, S. E. (1996) The relationship of theory and practice in the acquisition of skill. In: P. Benner, C. A. Tanner and C. A. Chesla (eds), *Expertise in Nursing Practice: Caring, Clinical Judgement, and Ethics* (New York: Springer Verlag).

Fleming, V. E. (1998) Women-with-midwives-with-women: a model of interdependence, *Midwifery*, 14(3): 137–43.

Geirsson, R. T., Gardarsdóttir, G., Pálsson, G. and Bjarnadóttir, R. I. (2006) *Skýrsla frá faedingarskráningu fyrir árid 2005* [a report on the documentation of births in 2005, with an English summary] (Reykjavík: Landspitali University Hospital, Women's Department & Children's Clinic).

Hall, J. (2001) *Midwifery, Mind and Spirit: Emerging Issues of Care* (Oxford: Books for Midwives).

Hall, J. and Taylor, M. (2004) Birth and spirituality. In: S. Downe (ed.), *Normal Childbirth: Evidence and Debate* (Edinburgh: Churchill Livingstone).

Halldorsdottir, S. and Karlsdottir, S. I. (1996) Journeying through labour and delivery: perceptions of women who have given birth, *Midwifery*, 12(2): 48–61.

Halldorsson, M. (2003) *Health Care Systems in Transition: Iceland* (Copenhagen: WHO Regional Office for Europe on behalf of the European Observatory on Health Systems and Policies).

Harding, P. and Bindloss, J. (2004) *Iceland*, 5th edn (London: Lonely Planet Publications; www.lonelyplanet.com).

Hodnett, E. D. (2006a) Caregiver support for women during childbirth, *Cochrane Database of Systematic Reviews,* 2 (accessed 12 June 2006).

Hodnett, E. D. (2006b) Continuity of caregivers for care during pregnancy and childbirth, *Cochrane Database of Systematic Reviews,* 2 (accessed 12 June 2006).

Hodnett, E. D., Gates, S., Hofmeyr, G. J. and Sakala, C. (2006) Continuous support for women during childbirth, *Cochrane Database of Systematic Reviews,* 2 (accessed 12 June 2006).

Hunter, B. (2001) Emotion work in midwifery: a review of current knowledge, *Journal of Advanced Nursing,* 34(4): 436–44.

Hunter, B. (2004) Conflicting ideologies as a source of emotion work in midwifery. *Midwifery,* 20(3): 261–72.

Hunter, B. (2005) Emotion work and boundary maintenance in hospital-based midwifery, *Midwifery,* 21(3): 253–66.

Johns, C. (2000) *Becoming a Reflective Practitioner: A Reflective and Holistic Approach to Clinical Nursing, Practice, Development, and Clinical Supervision* (Oxford: Blackwell).

Johns, C. (2002) *Guided Reflection: Advancing Practice* (Oxford: Blackwell Science).

Jónasson, J. (1961) *Íslenskir thjodhaettir* [Icelandic folkways and customs], 3rd edn (Reykjavík: Ísafoldarprentsmidja).

Jordan, B. (1997) Authoritative knowledge and its construction. In: R. E. Davis-Floyd and C. Sargent (eds), *Childbirth and Authoritative Knowledge: Cross-cultural Perspectives* (Berkeley, CA: University of California Press).

King, L. and Appleton, J. V. (1997) Intuition: a critical review of the research and rhetoric. *Journal of Advanced Nursing,* 26(1): 194–202.

Kirkham, M. (1997) Stories and childbirth. In: M. Kirkham and E. R. Perkins (eds), *Reflections on Midwifery* (London: Bailliere Tindall), pp.183–204.

Kirkham, M. (2000) How can we relate? In: M. Kirkham (ed.), *The Midwife–Mother Relationship* (Basingstoke: Palgrave Macmillan), pp. 227–54.

Kirkham, M. and Stapleton, H. (2000) Midwives' support needs as childbirth changes, *Journal of Advanced Nursing,* 32(2): 465–72.

Leap, N. (2000) The less we do, the more we give. In: M. Kirkham (ed.), *The Midwife–Mother Relationship* (Basingstoke: Palgrave Macmillan), pp. 1–18.

Leap, N. and Edwards, L. N. (2006) The politics of involving women in decision making. In: L. A. Page and R. McCandlish (eds), *The New Midwifery: Science and Sensitivity in Practice,* 2nd edn (Edinburgh: Churchill Livingstone), pp. 97–124.

Mander, R. (2001) *Supportive Care and Midwifery* (Oxford: Blackwell Science).

Ólafsdóttir, O. A. (2006) An Icelandic midwifery saga – Coming to light: 'With woman' and connective ways of knowing. Unpublished PhD thesis, Thames Valley University, London.

Page, L. (1993) Redefining the midwife role: changes needed in practice, *British Journal of Midwifery,* 1(1): 21–4.

Page, L. A. (2000) Keeping birth normal. In: *The New Midwifery: Science and Sensitivity in Practice,* 1st edn, ed. L. Page and P. Percival (Edinburgh: Churchill Livingstone).

Page, L. A. (2004) Working with women in childbirth. Unpublished PhD dissertation, University of Technology, Sydney.

Page, L. A. and McCandlish, R., eds (2006) *The New Midwifery: Science and Sensitivity in Practice*, 2nd edn (Edinburgh: Churchill Livingstone).

Pairman, S. (2006) Midwifery partnership working with women. In: L. A. Page and R. McCandlish (eds), *The New Midwifery: Science and Sensitivity in Practice*, 2nd edn (Edinburgh: Churchill Livingstone), pp. 73–97.

Polkinghorne, D. E. (1995) Narrative configuration in qualitative analysis. In: J. A. Hatch and R. Wisniewski (eds), *Life History and Narrative* (London: Falmer Press), pp. 5–24.

Sauls, D. J. (2002) Effects of labor support on mothers, babies, and birth outcomes, *Journal of Obstetric, Gynaecologic, and Neonatal Nursing*, 31(6): 733–41.

Siddiqui, J. (1999) Practice issues: the therapeutic relationship in midwifery, *British Journal of Midwifery*, 7(2): 111–14.

Siddiqui, J. (2005) The role of knowledge in midwifery decision making. In: M. D. Raynor, J. E. Marshall and A. Sullivan (eds), *Decision Making in Midwifery Practice* (New York: Churchill Livingstone), pp. 23–35.

Sigurðardóttir, A. (1984) Úr veröld kvenna – barnsburdur [From the world of women: giving birth]. In: B. Einarsdóttir (ed.), *Ljósmaedur á Íslandi II* (Reykjavík: Ljósmaedrafélag Íslands), pp. 137–311.

Statistics Iceland (2008) *Population* [online] (Reykjavík: Hagstofa Íslands (Statistics Iceland; available from: http://www.statice.is/?pageid=1175&src=/temp_en/mannfjoldi/faeddir.asp> (accessed: March 2008).

Vincent-Priya, J. (1991) *Birth without Doctors: Conversations with Traditional Midwives* (London: Earthscan Publications).

Wickham, S. (2004) Feminism and ways of knowing. In: M. Steward (ed.), *Pregnancy, Birth and Maternity Care* (Edinburgh: Books for Midwives), pp.157–68.

12

Peeling Onions: Using Drama to Explore Emotion

Kirsten Baker

Introduction

To be able to rehearse the areas of life which matter the most in a separate moment of time is a rare luxury. Novelists can do it on behalf of their fictional characters, but in real life the opportunities are rare. Like children playing, theatre allows us to replay and create moments of our own existence, both real and imagined. By harnessing different aspects of 'real' and 'pretend' we can explore and develop our emotional imagination, examining old territories and discovering new. Playing is not the same as being: it is *exploring* being.

Theatre is an embodied art form: human interactions, and interactions between individuals and context, are portrayed in theatre as events with a physical, spatial and aural reality. Theatrical (re)productions are designed to generate a response in the observers. Relationships, feelings and behaviours are always at the core of theatre practice. The capacity to use theatre consciously to explore these in the context of health care is what will be discussed in this chapter.

My own involvement with this praxis is apparent in this account. Professionally, I moved from being an actress to being a midwife, and now combine both in Progress Theatre, a midwifery theatre company. What Progress aims to do is bring the attributes of theatre into the culture of midwifery, allowing midwives to observe, analyse, debate and reinvent aspects of their own professional behaviours. The work is based on forum theatre, which was developed by Augusto Boal, a South American dramaturge who in turn based his work on that of Paolo Freire. The central tenets of Freire's *Pedagogy of the Oppressed* (1970) are that in contexts where oppressive behaviour dominates, it will be reproduced, and secondly, that liberation from oppression must be done *by* and not *on* those experiencing it. These both lie at the heart of Boal's work, and that of Progress Theatre.

Power: managing the emotions of others

Compared with other creative arts, the capacity to explore and even change feelings appears to be particularly associated with drama, and implicit in this is that it is the interactive nature of drama which enhances the 'real life' interactions. Because it is relationship-based, drama invokes overt and covert explorations of power between individuals, roles and contexts. An example of how this has been used in health-care practitioner education is the use of simulated patients in a way similar to the use of a mechanical simulator in a skills lab. Within this model, training sessions aimed at learning 'emotion-handling skills' is undertaken with standardised patients (for example, Yoo and Yoo 2003; Hannah et al. 2004).

In such a session, actors are briefed to portray the symptoms, attitudes and possible responses of a small number of particular patients. The health care professional then interacts with the 'patient' in a simulated consultation. This can be for training purposes, to rehearse skills in eliciting information, or to be exposed to potentially risky situations such as angry patients in a safe and controlled environment. Standardised patients are sometimes also in assessment.

There are a number of issues that arise from using 'pretend' in this way in order for health professionals to learn their role, and particularly about the role emotions play. First, the briefing of the 'patients' is congruent with a centrally agreed narrative. This in turn sits within the curriculum or training needs: the 'patients' are designed to help students meet specific learning objectives. This therefore begs the question of what attributes are seen as desirable in the emergent or developing professional. The ability to read, decode or even pre-empt the feelings and responses of others emerges as a fairly key skill.

In this type of simulation, where decoding the patient is the aim, the 'real' and 'pretend' qualities of the interaction can be seen as a kind of code-breaking exercise. By dissecting the encounter, the health professional can learn about what makes this particular patient respond and react in particular ways. The patient becomes the subject of a study to the professionals' gaze – but with no autonomy or independence of voice. It may therefore be perilously easy to move from the particular to the general. The goal here is arguably to produce clinicians who behave appropriately according to overt and covert professional codes – adept at managing the emotions of others.

Thus, within this use of simulation, both pedagogically and clinically the power resides almost entirely with the professional. The managing of emotions deepens even further the distribution of power, and harnessing real and pretend to this end reinforces this discourse.

There are other ways of using drama to delve into the encounter between health care practitioners and those they care for. These can be less neat, and have a less 'managerial' content.

'I was just being me': encountering emotional complexity using drama

Julie had not felt her baby move for several days – although she couldn't be completely sure. When her mother suggested she should go and see the midwife, she knew she was right – and she also knew why she had been avoiding doing so. It turned out to be every bit as dreadful as she had feared: the midwife, Carrie, was as gentle as she could be, but there was no escaping the look on her face as she moved the heart monitor over Julie's jelly-smeared abdomen in ever-decreasing circles.

As Carrie turned to Julie, her guts heaved as the reality of the silence where the baby's heartbeat should have been heard filled the room. It was not the first time: this time, though, she felt her capacity to cope slipping. She turned to her colleagues and said, 'I don't know what to say'. In real life, she had never been able to do this: her duty of care meant she could not fall apart – not until afterwards anyway. It was also the first time that the encounter had been shared with her colleagues as it was actually happening. Despite this, it felt extraordinarily real: she could access her real grief, despair and rage at what had happened. She also felt unnervingly 'unskilled'.

This meeting between Julie and Carrie occurred in a place that was fraught with intense emotions, uncertainty and threatened roles. This was real. However, it took place in a 'pretend' clinic, in an artificial setting and time. The two of them began by pretending to be alone, though in reality they were being watched by a group of Carrie's colleagues, also keen to explore this uncomfortable terrain within the safety of pretend. Julie was actually Sue, an actress taking the part of Julie – pretending – while Carrie was 'playing with' her own role: that of the midwife. They were participating in a drama-based workshop to explore breaking bad news. This differed from the learning of skills: rather, it engaged the health care professional in a potentially troubling encounter with her own emotional turmoil.

Although tearful, Carrie persisted in reflecting on her own feelings and performance. Using structured feedback, she was encouraged to identify what she did well. Her colleagues too were asked for their feedback, and one said that she felt that Carrie was professionally skilled at giving accurate information about how the procedure around a confirmed fetal death would proceed.

Sue, still in role as Julie, could also reflect on what was happening: as she heard this information she felt uneasy. She did not doubt that the 'induction' that she heard Carrie talking about would be done in a completely professional manner. On some level, too, she knew that the information being offered would be invaluable at some point. The truth, however, was that she had heard little of Carrie's explanation of the clinical procedure. 'I'm not sure that's what I want to hear right now', she explained to Carrie and her colleagues, 'my heart wasn't really into hearing about it . . .'

Carrie listened carefully. She realised that *her* heart wasn't really in that clinical explanation either, however smoothly she delivered it. She just felt she ought to do it; ought to offer some professional advice or information in the face of the bleak reality. It was something she *could* talk about: relatively safe territory in the vastness of sadness and uncertainty.

Her realisation seemed transformative. What happened at this point in the learning was beyond the models, assumptions and information she already had: it was what she didn't know. This seemed crucial.

This appeared to offer her an opportunity for *un*learning, or for abandoning the domain which was familiar and which she had never been able to leave before. Gradually, they built up from this place of unlearning. Using the patient's experiences as a touchstone, she was able to stay very closely with her own feelings and experiences. As the interaction was resumed, she fed these into her responses to Julie.

Afterwards, reflecting on what had happened, Carrie made an interesting observation: she said she forgot about being a midwife and 'I was just being me'. This distinction between the professional role and the visceral experience of caring suggests that, from Carrie's point of view, the uncomfortable feelings invoked by the encounter sat at odds with her perception of herself as a professional.

Reality and pretend

For Carrie and her colleagues, experiences that were 'real', 'imagined', 'pretend' and 'playing' jostled and shifted alongside each other, mobilising what appeared to be high levels of reflection and learning. To Carrie, the consultation felt very real: for the most part she was not aware of being observed. However, it was simultaneously not real in particular ways. First, the simulation meant the midwife was freed from the responsibility to look after the woman. Uniquely, the entire meeting would have no impact whatsoever on the woman and her feelings – because it was 'pretend'. An important part of such a simulation is the moment when the actress comes out of role: Julie leaves and Sue arrives. Secondly, it also meant that the insights of the patient both within what was happening, and reflecting on it afterwards in role, became an accessible part of the learning. The midwife usually imagines the perspective of the woman: here it was real; it was articulated and heard. Thirdly, the colleagues who watched were able to participate in the experience. They are not usually present in clinical encounters, and although reflections on practice may take place with peers, this will be based on an account of what happened rather than a shared presence.

The learning for the midwives was in an arena of professional practice which was both *familiar* and *uncomfortable*. The familiarity and discomfort can readily generate the feeling rules or 'socially structured defence mechanisms' (Menzies 1960:100) which have been discussed in other chapters within this book, especially Chapters 4 and 10.

Using drama in this way appears to have a number of benefits. First, by making a usually private encounter visible, it allows for a shared acknowledgement of the feelings it generates. They are put up to scrutiny, becoming part of the public space. Secondly, the client becomes a fellow explorer in the reflective process. This can dislodge any view that it is the patient, rather than the situation that is difficult. Thirdly, it can entail 'playing with' the professional role: temporarily moving outside of it into the 'personal' domain. By doing this, questions about the nature of professionalism can be raised: it can be a helpful way to reflect on what, exactly, we are putting on when we assume our professional role.

Playing can be both risky and safe. It can involve an experience of powerlessness in the face of some of the uncertainties implicit in difficult aspects of care. Part of the attempt to manage uncertainty may be to try to convert aspects of the 'case' into observable, measurable behaviours which can be reproduced. In the session where Julie met Carrie, the aim was not to teach professional tricks or devices for managing patients: in some ways Carrie's notion of being 'skilled' was being challenged. By allowing what was happening to open up her own vulnerability rather than prompting a delivery of a professional response, she was able to be and stay alongside Julie most effectively. The value and meaning of this sort of professional relationship has been explored by Berg et al. (1996) and by Anderson (2000).

Personal experience: making progress

As well as being hugely challenging for the midwife, this work was also so for Sue, the actress playing Julie. With no script or rehearsals, the often powerful encounters played out in this way emerged moment by moment, both participants feeling their way within their respective roles. But while Sue was acting – or pretending – for Carrie it was her own role she was playing.

It was through working as an actress in workshops such as this one that I became interested in becoming a midwife. It was a privilege over the years to observe and participate as health professionals grappled with the emotional content of some of their encounters. My fascination with health care providers grew, and I decided to cross the professional Rubicon. I became a midwife in 1994.

Having entered the profession with this background, it was a shock as I began my own clinical work to observe how marginalised women's experiences seemed sometimes to be. Working long shifts without a break ground us all down. It pitted midwife against midwife, and midwife against client, for it was they, surely, who stood in the way of decent working conditions. This was a particularly difficult pill to swallow, since my route into professional health care practice had been through my experience, as an actress, of articulating the patient voice. Them and us: we now seemed to be on opposite sides of the divide. I was torn in two.

I knew what I was doing often fell far short of even the lowest acceptable standard of care. With the last vestiges of my motivation I dragged myself off to study days. These confirmed my experience that what we were doing was not good enough. 'Do it better' seemed to be the message. 'Promote normal birth' better; 'Detect child abuse' better; 'Document' better. We returned to work unchanged. This distance between the rhetoric of care and its delivery was perplexing. None of us set out to 'care' so inadequately, and the cost of doing so seemed often to be high. Serendipitously an opportunity to develop Progress Theatre emerged from this gloom, involving other midwives and an actor with experience in forum theatre.

In 1998 Mavis Kirkham took part in a forum theatre workshop exploring issues of domestic violence. The project was commissioned by Sheffield Men Against Violence in partnership with Theatreworks, of which Bill McDonnell was a long-standing member. The way in which this methodology drew the spectators into analysis of familiar dilemmas seemed to offer huge potential for midwifery learning. There were also parallels with the sort of interactive drama work in which I was involved and which has been described above.

Following a meeting between Mavis, Bill and myself, the idea of using forum theatre within midwifery education began to take shape. We recruited other midwives and drama practitioners, and began by starting to find out about how student midwives experienced clinical work through focus groups and workshops. Our first show, *How was It for You?*, was the result.

In showing this to the students, and asking them to engage with the material, there seemed to be an arena for reflection, recognition, analysis and debate. We went on to devise and present more shows: *I Don't Know How She Got Pregnant* looks at the impact and implications of caring for women who have been sexually abused; *Fixing It* deals with drug-abusing women; *Swimming in Concrete* with workplace culture, pressures and bullying at work; and *Every3Days* with domestic abuse. At the heart of each of these, and in the workshops that accompany them, is the experience of midwives and others at work. The format allows for close and detailed observation of real working situations, and allows the possibility to comment on and perhaps change what occurs. In multi-agency fora, a further layer is added where the routines and practices of different professional groups can be shared across agencies. Areas where words are shared, but where understanding may differ, can be made visible: examples may include routine enquiry, referral and assessment.

In this the work differs from some of the study days I attended, whose starting point was the work itself, and the deficiencies of midwives in not doing it well enough. The reason for the approach that Progress Theatre takes is twofold. First, based on the analysis of Paulo Freire (1970), the foundation of the pedagogic method should be the learner rather than the notional 'lesson'. Secondly, as members of Progress Theatre we believe in the principle of parallel processes: that is to say, if midwives are valued (and learn to value themselves) more highly, they in turn will have the capacity to value those for whom they care more highly.

In the ten years since its inception there have been changes in the group membership, but the work is essentially as it was then: devising short shows on the basis of our own and others' experiences of being midwives, and then using performance and a drama-based workshop to harness the audience – consisting also of those closely involved in maternity care – to explore their actions, reactions, feelings and behaviour within their workplace, and the influence these all have on each other.

There is an underlying analysis that the feelings and behaviour of individuals are strongly linked to context. This is crucial if the work of Progress Theatre is to help midwives move beyond a sense of victimhood into a more politicised perspective. This experience of oppression arguably has its roots in the system by which midwifery is and has been shaped: indeed it could be seen as historically logical for it to be as it is (Kirkham 1999). The argument of Progress Theatre, however, is that it is not inevitable. Progress Theatre seeks to present to midwives this world both 'as it is and as capable of transformation' (Boal 1979: 132).

How was it for you?

A Progress Theatre workshop opens with a theatrical performance of clinical midwifery life. Although the script becomes fixed, we start by improvising, or devising. Devising is an established theatre technique, designed to produce material by actors improvising from within their own experiences. This method is appropriate for the work since we are using high levels of reflexivity and reconstruction of our own stories: it also means that the emotions experienced by the characters are close to those portraying them – most of whom are midwives.

As the initial scenes unfold, with some of the excesses of midwifery behaviour heightened for comedic effect, midwives in the audience can be seen reacting with a mixture of horror and fascination. They laugh, too, but this does not seem to diminish their sense of identification with what they see: a frequent comment afterwards is, 'Did you base this on our Unit?'

We then use a technique whereby the audience is invited to watch the scenes again, and can give their interpretation of what the characters are thinking or feeling at any one time. Known as 'Stop! Think!' the technique freezes the action, enabling characters to talk about what is happening beneath the surface of their conduct. Boal states that '[it] is specifically designed to seek out the internal truth of each person, the hidden truth, the unformulated things . . .' (Boal 1995: 175). The exercise is in effect an invitation to express any such insights both *on* and *in* the action: a very conscious summons to articulate and reflect on the feelings generated by the social interactions portrayed. In doing so it is also evoking feelings, thoughts and behaviour in conjunction with each other.

When used in psychodrama this technique is called 'doubling': once again, it allows for those *watching* a scene to engage with what the characters *within* the scene are thinking and feeling – scenes which are based on participants' experiences. The basis for responses is their *own* identification with what is happening.

Such a deconstruction highlights the fact that overt behaviours and their emotional content may be different. It also allows for a perception that moves beyond judgement towards empathy. This is complex: identifying with the inner feelings of a bullying member of staff, for example, may seem to be condoning the behaviour by sympathising with the motivation. However, in moving towards recognising the emotional terrain beneath such behaviours, there may be benefit in exposing, demystifying and possibly diffusing its power. The acknowledgement of this terrain is an important component in the development of emotional intelligence (Hunter 2004).

As the scene resumes, the action can be taken in different directions at the suggestion of those watching. New material, interactions and feelings can be generated in improvised scenes. Louise, for example, is initially portrayed as a collusive bully-in-the-making who, through her actions and inactions, makes the experience of a more recent member of staff bleaker and even more marginalised. The audience suggest how she might behave differently, and are invited to come and take her place to demonstrate their proposed change. What changes could be implemented – and what may ensue – can be a springboard for much debate about what feelings motivate and result from different behaviours, and can invoke high levels of 'reflection on and reflection in action' (Schön 1983). It can also signify an exciting dissolution of any distinction between actors and audience, and between real and pretend.

Feelings and contexts

What has been described here so far is very much the internal landscape of individual feelings. Relationships between individuals, and between individual and context, can also be given physical, spatial and aural form using space and imagination. In a Progress Theatre workshop, this ensues from the initial presentation of scenes and takes one of the characters portrayed as a starting point. Starting with, for example, Sarah, the 'joker'[1] asks what is the most important factor – or relationship – influencing her experience. Words like 'hassle', 'pressure', 'making her unhappy' are often used to describe Sarah's experiences of the clinical environment: what emerges in this relationship is highly emotionally charged. This exercise unfurls gradually as the participants work out how to engage with the material. The joker quite deliberately does not give extensive instructions, but responds to comments from those watching, and slowly they are drawn from commenting on to participating in the action. Once suggestions are made about what is impacting on Sarah – and these may differ and be debated – the joker encourages another member of the audience to show *how* it is impacting. A heavy workload, for example, may be shown by someone pressing down on Sarah's shoulders, literally weighing her down. Similarly 'paperwork' may be physically demonstrated by a person fluttering their hands in front of Sarah's face; 'management' as someone standing behind and above her. The audience chooses, and part of what emerges is their own experience – of endless form-filling or policy directives, for example. They are asked about other relationships; these are portrayed using the same technique, and gradually the confidence and skill of the spectators grows. They begin to make suggestions by demonstrating with their bodies: 'Like this', they say, as they adopt a pose, and with each addition more of the emotional landscape is exposed to view. As uncomfortable as the subject matter is, there is much hilarity as Sarah's full bladder steps onto the stage, following an observation that this is a highly significant factor for her well-being!

By giving such experiences physical form, we are touching on the physicality of feelings, and the emotion memories held in our bodies. Bodies and minds, like thoughts and feelings, are sometimes held as dualities: here they are integrated and incorporated with each other.

'Spect-acting'

Theatre practitioners have since time immemorial harnessed the relationship between real and pretend, creating and playing with the shadows such a relationship can throw up in different ways and to different effect. Part of what happens in the exercise described above is that relationships are disrupted: the audience become part of the performance, and the actors become bystanders as their audience take the stage. Boal coined a particular word – spectactor – to describe this confounding of categories. How Boal came to develop this particular relationship is interesting, as it raises important issues about owner-ship and oppression, both of which underpin much of the emotional toxicity of organisations and work to address it (Deery and Kirkham 2007).

The relationship between the actors and spectators intrigued Boal as it had done dramaturges from Aristotle to Brecht and beyond. In this relationship he saw important power issues between the 'doers' and the 'done to'. After several years of devising and performing plays which, in essence, showed oppressed people their experience and demonstrated a solution, he was brought to a new realisation, and it was from this that the notion of the 'spectactor' was born. Boal tells (Boal 1995) of how this came about, one evening after a performance in which the actors had portrayed the righteous and violent overthrow of an oppressive landlord. This, as usual, was greeted rapturously, and after the applause died down at the end of the show, a member of the audience rushed up to Boal with a suggestion. Many of the people gathered there were proposing to undertake such a raid that very night, and Boal and the company were sure to want to come along – weren't they? Boal patiently explained that what they did as actors was not to actually perform any actions they showed (particularly the risky ones) but to explain to others what actions they should be taking. This was greeted somewhat frostily, and Boal began to rethink his use of theatre.

The company evolved so that instead of showing problems and proposed solutions, they showed dilemmas and invited the audience to suggest a solution. He coined the word 'to difficultate' – this can be a messy process where the aim, unlike that of facilitation, may not be to tie up and neaten any loose threads. It is also much more emotionally vivid, as the content of the drama is spontaneously provoked, with a strong sense of ownership by those watching.

Boal's work developed further after another seminal encounter. After showing a difficult problem between a husband and wife, the audience were asked for their suggestions as to how to proceed. As the suggestions were made, the actors portrayed them amongst much discussion and analysis about the behaviours and feelings of those involved. Boal noticed, however, that one member of the audience, a woman who had repeatedly made a suggestion about what should happen, was looking deeply dissatisfied with what was being acted out. Eventually, and with some exasperation, Boal invited the woman to show exactly what it was that she wanted to see: 'If you are still not satisfied, why don't you come on stage yourself and show us what you mean' (Boal 1995: 6). She did so.

This is important in terms of whose emotional territory is being explored. Again, there are important overlaps between forum theatre and psychodrama (Feldhendler 1994) in terms of the impact this level of engagement this can have on an individual's emotional literacy, and their capacity to challenge and change previously held 'truths' about themselves.

Essentially, while forum theatre addresses social inequalities, and the experience of the individual within that, psychodrama takes a more individual and psychotherapeutic approach. Both, however, are centred on the experience of the protagonist whose story is depicted. In each case, the function of the ensuing actions and interactions is to explore and rebuild potentially painful or limiting experiences, and the circumstances that may have brought these about. New experiences may be incorporated by being acted out, and a new emotional repertoire can be established.

Central to this is the idea of schemas, or cognitive structures (Beck 1967). These are in essence the existing emotional patterns held by an individual which direct or dictate behaviour. Drama is seen as a highly effective way of manifesting and working with these schemas, activating them with great intensity and in context (Padesky 1994). It also has the potential to 'provide a powerful first experience of what it would be like for the client to hold a different schema and respond to events and others in new ways' (Padesky 1994: 277). This echoes Boal's notion that forum theatre can adduce new concepts of self and behaviour.

Conclusion

Using drama within health care may be particularly apt because of the dissonance between the emotional content of much of our work and the organisational structures within which we provide it (Hunter and Deery 2005). As we hurtle through the 'normal' emotional roller-coaster of our days, we may – or may not – have time to reflect on and untangle the substance of our actions and interactions.

Drama has the potential to provide a space and a trigger to allow for such reflections to take place with intensity and in safety. It also allows for the simultaneous mobilisation of the rational, cognitive domain with the affective domain. The perceived dualities between thoughts and feelings, bodies and minds can be dissolved. For this engagement to be effective, what happens needs to feel sufficiently real to be meaningful, and sufficiently pretend to allow for the reality to be safely played with.

The ways in which drama plays with our reality will, as in any relationship-based practice, embody issues of power and control. It also engages bodies and minds in the exploration of feeling for, as Augusto Boal says, 'the human being is a unity, and indivisible whole . . . A bodily movement "is" a thought and a thought expresses itself in corporeal form' (Boal 1992: 61).

Reflective questions

1   Where do you think feelings 'live'?

2   To what extent does working in an institution govern your feelings?

3   Name the feelings associated with going against the system?

Note

1   Boal coined this word (as in a 'wild card') to describe the director, or facilitator/ difficultator of the group process.

References

Anderson, T. (2000) Feeling safe enough to let go: the relationship between a woman and her midwife during the second stage of labour. In: M. Kirkham (ed.), *The Midwife–Mother Relationship* (Basingstoke: Palgrave Macmillan).

Beck, A. T. (1967) *Depression: Clinical, Experimental and Theoretical Aspects* (New York: Harper & Row).

Berg, M., Lundgren, I., Hermansson, E. and Wahlberg, V. (1996) Women's experience of the encounter with the midwife during childbirth, *Midwifery*, 12: 11–15.

Boal, A. (1979) *Theatre of the Oppressed* (London: Pluto).

Boal, A. (1992) *Games for Actors and Non Actors* (London: Routledge).

Boal, A. (1995) *The Rainbow of Desire: The Boal Method of Theatre and Therapy* (London: Routledge).

Deery, R. and Kirkham, M. (2007) Drained and dumped on: the generation and accumulation of emotional toxic waste in community midwifery. In: M. Kirkham (ed.), *Exploring the Dirty Side of Women's Health* (London: Routledge).

Feldhendler, D. (1994) Augusto Boal and Jacob Moreno: theatre and therapy. In: M. Schutzman and J. Cohen-Cruz (eds), *Playing Boal* (London: Routledge).

Freire, P. (1970) *Pedagogy of the Oppressed* (London: Penguin).

Hannah, A., Millichamp, C. J. and Ayers, K. M. (2004) A communication skills course for undergraduate dental students, *Journal of Dental Education*, 68(9): 970–7.

Hunter, B. (2004) The importance of emotional intelligence in midwifery. Editorial, *British Journal of Midwifery*, October, 12(10): 1–2.

Hunter, B. and Deery, R. (2005) Building our knowledge about emotion work in midwifery: combining and comparing findings from two different research studies, *Evidence Based Midwifery*, 3(1): 10–15.

Kirkham, M. (1999) Exclusion in maternity care. In: M. Purdy and D. Banks (eds), *Health and Exclusion* (London: Routledge).

Menzies, I. (1960) A case study in the functioning of social systems as a defence against anxiety, *Human Relations*, 13: 95–121.

Padesky, C. (1994) Schema change processes in cognitive therapy, *Clinical Psychology and Psychotherapy*, 1: 267–78.

Schön, D. (1983) *The Reflective Practitioner: How Professionals Think in Action* (New York: Basic Books).

Yoo, M. S. and Yoo, I. Y. (2003) The effectiveness of standardized patients as a teaching method for nursing fundamentals, *Journal of Nursing Education*, 42(10): 444–8.

Part IV
Weaving It All Together

13

Emotion Work around Reproduction: Supportive or Constraining?

Mavis Kirkham

This book explores the emotion work of women at key points in their reproductive life and the emotion work of their carers in their professional and personal reproductive lives. The concepts used have developed within the social sciences over a number of years.

Our management of emotions is grounded in our relationships and our social context. Feelings are socially constructed, even, or especially, those connected with reproduction. This is demonstrated in the differing personal presentations of the visceral, painful experience of labour; any study of birth in different places and at different times in history makes this abundantly clear. Feelings and associated behaviours are adjusted relative to social norms, the relative importance of relationships and fears of upsetting others.

Context and territory

Context largely determines the nature of most of our relationships. Glaser and Strauss described the 'sentimental order' of a hospital ward in 1968: 'the intangible but very real patterning of mood and sentiment that characteristically exists on a ward' (Glaser and Strauss 1968: 14). This order is very powerful. Though Glaser and Strauss studied death, I found the concept immensely useful when studying interaction on a consultant unit labour ward (Kirkham 1987). The smooth running of the medically controlled labour ward was all-important; doctors controlled the management of labour and its pain, midwives and mothers controlled behaviour and emotions to make the system work smoothly. This involved tight control of emotions on all sides to achieve 'the language and politeness of the labour ward which allowed a semblance of caring and concern whilst ignoring the needs unmet by the power system' (Kirkham 1987: 214). Mothers took their cues from midwives, while midwives were intent upon 'jollying women along the maternity trajectory that has been mapped out for them' (Edwards, Chapter 2). Such emotional labour achieves compliant, hierarchical working relationships as described by Ruth Deery in Chapter 4.

As early as 1980 Ann Thompson observed of midwives, 'We have become assembly line workers . . .' (Thompson 1980: 68). This has been echoed in many subsequent studies. Fiona Dykes's recent research (Chapter 5 and Dykes 2006) was on postnatal wards, traditionally regarded as midwives' territory, but situated within the overall 'medical production line' of the hospital. Production-line work creates feelings of alienation (Marx 1887), especially with increasing workloads (Seigrist 1996) and powerlessness (Seligman 1975). It also produces coping mechanisms which can be emotionally 'damaging rather than edifying' (Chapter 2), leading in the long term to burnout (Sandall 1997,1998).

Not all settings identified with women's reproductive health fit the conveyor-belt image, nor are they all experienced as medical territory (see Chapters 1, 11 and 12). In my early study, what was then termed 'the GP Unit' was the midwives' territory and the home was the territory of the family. In both these settings labour and its pain could not be medically controlled so co-operation was evident and feelings displayed in such ways as to support the woman coping with her labour. This has been demonstrated more recently in Denis Walsh's ethnographic study of a free standing birth-centre. This birth centre was clearly the midwives' territory and they worked continuously, 'honing the birth environment' to create 'a friendly calm atmosphere' (Walsh 2006a: 232) Such 'environmental nurture' was evident in the setting and in the behaviour of the staff who sought to 'comfort and protect' women in labour and pamper and make them feel special postnatally. Such nurturing of the 'becoming mother' is conceptualised as 'matrescence', which 'seems to tread a delicate path between listening, talking, showing, observing and leaving alone' (p. 237). To achieve such subtle emotional care and concentration on the cues given by the mother, the midwife herself must have a degree of autonomy and control of her working environment. Matrescence is not compatible with the processing required in hospital, or with the feeling that midwives' work is closely monitored. In many ways it resembles care of mother and baby by a grandmother: care given with love by someone who knows how motherhood feels and respects the autonomy of her daughter.

Autonomy

Relationships with clients and colleagues are key sources of job satisfaction for midwives and the state of these relationships plays an important part in midwives' decisions to stay or to leave midwifery (Kirkham et al. 2006). Emotional labour is carried out through relationships. Where the aim of emotional labour is to ensure client compliance, strict emotional discipline is called for, whether the setting is that of an airliner (Hochschild 1983), or a smoothly run ward or clinic. The fundamental aim in these settings is emotional processing so that clients feel safe, behave in the 'right' way and feel positive about the experience with minimal investment of precious staff time. What is 'right' behaviour is not decided by the practitioners on the ground. In these settings, staff have little autonomy or freedom to decide where to invest their time. The necessary 'deep acting' (Hochschild 1983) earns no appreciation or applause, but carries a personal toll as the continuing 'holding in' (Deery, Chapter 4) of the midwife's feelings is draining, alienating and damaging in the long run. The 'regulatory, coercive aspects of emotional labour as it is played out by health practitioners' (Edwards, Chapter 2) or the need to 'curtail patient demands' (Bone, Chapter 3) may prove emotionally corrosive in the long run for those practitioners, manifesting in high occupational stress. Long practice in these aspects of emotional labour certainly limits their repertoire of professional, emotional response.

Where staff have more autonomy, they are more generous in their relationships and can facilitate autonomy in their clients. This has been found in medicine (Kaplan et al. 1996) and in midwifery (see Chapter 1, Chapter 10; Hunter 2004, 2005, 2006). Such relative autonomy is usually found away from the closely monitored hospital setting and where professional and client have a continuing relationship rather than a single consultation. Here emotional labour is more complex and subtle. Where staff have a degree of freedom in their use of time, they may choose to 'invest time' early in a relationship (Deery, Chapter 4) to enhance a client's confidence and personal resources. Staff 'need time' and flexibility in their use of time 'in order to give time to others' (Dykes, Chapter 5). The giving of time and attention demonstrates that women are worth that attention and provides the opportunity for them to raise their concerns, rather than just being clinically 'checked'. Relationships thus become more balanced. Within that balance, midwives can facilitate the development of women's social support networks that will enhance their own and their community's social capital and enrich their lives postnatally (Leap 2000). Such balanced relationships also mean that midwives can experience clients as supporting them (see Chapter 10), rather than feeling an unremitting one-way drain of emotional energy (Deery and Kirkham 2007).

Several chapters in this book describe how midwives can create an atmosphere of calm which is reassuring for a labouring women (e.g. Chapters 10 and 11). This may involve skilful acting, to avoid alarming the parents (see Chapter 10) but it is usually a source of professional pride for midwives and confidence for their clients (see Chapter 11). Where this is the case, relationships remain professional but can become two-way: mutually respectful and considerate. Creating an atmosphere of calm is a major achievement in hospital but easier where midwives have more control of their work setting (e.g. Walsh, 2006a, 2006b).

Similarly, colleague relationships are often neglected under pressures towards conformity in large, hierarchical structures. When staff work with small groups of trusted colleagues, relationships can be sustaining and enabling (Chapter 1 and Kirkham 2003).

Reciprocity

Table 1.1 shows very clearly the potential of reciprocal relationships in maternity care. 'Being a person not a role' improves the quality of any relationship and the benefits for mothers and midwives are clearly stated. This is possible because these relationships develop over time where both parties adjust to each other as individuals and the midwives have a degree of autonomy in managing their work. Such quality of care and of relationship has been demonstrated in many settings where there is continuity of care and it is not coincidental that these are often out of hospital settings. Even for women needing hospital care, the experience of mother and midwife is very different if care, on what is otherwise a conveyor belt, is provided by a known midwife who is there for this particular consultation, rather than to provide fragmented care to many unknown women.

With continuity of care the loyalty of midwives shifts from institution and profession towards clients (Chapter 1). This is logical since relationships with clients now form a continuing and important part of the midwife's life rather than short encounters in a professional life which is dominated by relationships with other professionals. Emotional investment can be made in relationships which are ongoing, rather than transitory, with benefit for both parties. Mander (2001) brought together research on midwifery and on support and concluded that supportive relationships are reciprocal and constitute a social exchange. So many studies have demonstrated midwives' desire for support (e.g. Stapleton et al. 1998; Kirkham and Stapleton 2001; Deery 2005), yet so much of their work is experienced as emotionally draining rather than in any way restoring their emotional resources or giving satisfaction (e.g. Deery and Kirkham 2007). In Chapter 8 Chris Bewley demonstrates how support for midwives who had experienced pregnancy loss had to be appropriate to them as individuals rather than formulaic and possibly hurtful. Such support 'was sometimes consequent on a degree of self-disclosure, with its attendant risks'. This is true between colleagues and between professionals and clients; risky self-disclosure can occur more easily in relationships where the other person has proved herself to be trustworthy, and this takes time.

Safety and trust

We feel safe where we trust our setting and the people around us. Many health service users have described their relationships with health professionals in ways which show how they link trust with safety (e.g. Kirkham and Stapleton 2001; Edwards 2005). Walsh describes a 'mothering' dimension to birth centre care which makes women feel safe, and demonstrates the 'complex weave of physical, psychological and cultural and social dimensions of safety' (Walsh 2006a: 236). To be useful, health services have to be based upon assumptions of trust and safety. Nurses and midwives put a great deal of invisible, unacknowledged emotional work into establishing and maintaining services which are perceived as caring and trustworthy (e.g. Chapters 3 and 11). Yet fragmented relationships within a pressurised, industrialised model of care do not allow for the development of trust and can undermine perceptions of safety. Here again, time is crucial. Fiona Dykes describes women 'subjected to superficial, formal, intermittent and time-pressured encounters at a time when they were emotionally vulnerable and lacking in confidence with breastfeeding' (Chapter 5). She argues that hospital may be seen as a place of safety should something 'go wrong', but for women seeking support in a major life transition and learning new skills in breastfeeding 'it is not emotionally safe'.

The emotional work of professionals within hospital is doubly frustrating because it is invisible and unacknowledged and, though essential, it works against the grain of the organisation which is one of control rather than trust and relationship. Emotional work in such a setting is bound to be more concerned with ensuring clinical control and compliance than with individualised care and facilitation. As such it cannot give the rewards of reciprocal relationship, though clients are perceptive and may be considerate in deciding not to 'trouble' the midwife with their problems.

Where women perceive that midwives trust their ability to birth their baby, this trust is experienced as enabling (Lundgren and Dahlberg 1998; Edwards 2005). It is also a source of professional pride for the midwife (Walsh 2006a, 2006b). Pressures of time and standardisation of care make it difficult for hospital midwives to trust women's ability to give birth normally and perceptions of trust and calm can be lost when care is fragmented.

Coping with the care deficit

Whilst there is ample evidence that relationships that are supportive and caring improve clinical outcomes (Halldorsdóttir and Karlsdóttir 1996; Hodnett 2002), these aspects of modern health care are low in status, if not invisible (Bone, Chapter 3; Murphy-Lawless 1998). The privileging of technology over care is evident throughout health care and much of the discourse of modern nursing and midwifery demonstrates how status comes with technical rather than caring work. If time is limited, it is the technical rather than the caring work which must be done. Arlie Russell Hochschild speaks of a 'care deficit in both private and public life' (Hochschild 2003: 214). Debora Bone describes nurses 'needing to curtail patient demands to match nurses' diminished availability' (Chapter 3). In an industrial model of care, it is as true of British midwifery as it is of American nursing that women 'learn to do without' emotional support in labour. 'The social context – the care deficit – is culturally transformed into a psychological issue: "Can I manage my emotional needs to match the minimalist norms of care?"' (Hochschild 2003: 221). In maternity care such questions are answered by providing pain relief rather than supporting women in coping with pain in labour, and the emotional work undertaken by staff is that which ensures compliance with the norms of client behaviour. Childbearing women are dependent on busy midwives and 'don't like to ask' for their needs to be met in consideration of their midwives' busyness. So both sides withdraw from the relationship. This cannot be useful preparation of the great relational and emotional demands of parenthood.

Detachment has often been seen as a professional attribute, the professional identifying with a body of knowledge and practice, rather than individual patients. The tension between this model of professionalism and the tradition of caring and being 'with woman' has long been felt by nurses and midwives. Recent trends towards a more industrialised model of care based on cost-saving business economics have led to other manifestations of detachment. Susan Battersby, in Chapter 6, describes the emotional labour of attributing 'otherness': a means by which midwives distance themselves from mothers and colleagues whose behaviour has the potential to cause them distress. Such labelling usually carries blame and maintains a culture in which stereotyping is all too common (Kirkham et al. 2002a). It is a way of coping that creates division between colleagues (Curtis et al. 2006) and between staff and clients. Reasons for behaviour are not considered and such blaming ensures that relationships are superficial and, as they are prevented from producing negative emotions, they cannot be worked upon to become positive or rewarding. Relationships with colleagues are crucial to midwives' job satisfaction (Kirkham et al. 2006), yet the attribution of 'otherness' divides colleagues and limits their relationships. It also creates situations where much emotional labour is expended on endeavouring to fit in, rather than discussing differences.

Pressures of time and lack of emotional skills beyond those of containment may account for the phenomenon of midwives 'checking not listening' to women (Edwards 2005; Kirkham et al. 2002b). Increasing tasks of monitoring and checking, without added resources, crowd out discussion and listening. Women may be processed to accept routinised care and to 'do without' their individual needs being heard, but it is at considerable cost to both parties. For groups of women who may be particularly vulnerable and anxious this is particularly important, as Helen Allan and Gina Finnerty demonstrate in Chapter 7. It also robs midwives of a fundamental source of job satisfaction.

Learning emotional skills

Because emotional labour isn't acknowledged or rewarded, it isn't taught and it has only recently been studied. However, it is closely observed by those new to a setting.

Billie Hunter describes how 'students learn "what midwives do" in relation to emotional display through trial and error' (Chapter 10), and 'mixed messages' thus abound. She sees 'affective neutrality' – the suppression of emotion to maintain a professional image – as more common in hospital and fitting with institutional goals. (Community midwives were more likely to adopt an approach of 'affective awareness'.) These students' suppression of emotion in order to fit in has a parallel in midwives returning to practice who prioritise 'appearing competent' in order to fit in with colleagues, though this may delay the development of real competence (Kirkham and Morgan 2006).

Billie Hunter also describes students learning to detach by 'switching off and toughening up' when circumstances felt overwhelming. Such self-protective responses are inevitable if there is no education or modelling of ways of processing and learning from difficult experiences. Self-protection is important but so often the coping strategies adopted may protect in the short term and damage in the long term (Menzies Lyth 1988), by having a negative impact on relationships with clients (see Chapter10) and limiting the potential for job satisfaction. Coping strategies range from small personal detachments to bullying, the impact of which is widespread and damaging (Kirkham et al. 2006; Kirkham 2007). Damaging coping strategies may be adopted for good reason, but they need to be changed just as much as the conditions which brought them about need to be changed, for the benefit of all concerned.

Women take their cues from midwives (Edwards, Chapter 2). So often staff cues are defensive and women learn not to raise emotional issues with them, but to behave in a detached manner themselves. In this respect women are very considerate towards their midwives and the emotional labour of midwives processing women is successful in achieving 'informed compliance' (Kirkham and Stapleton 2001). Positive examples of the learning of emotional skills can also be found in this book. In Chapter 1 Chris McCourt and Trudy Stevens describe how caseload midwives 'gained satisfaction and reward from their emotional relationships with women'. They state that 'a high level of autonomy in their practice, and the ability to form supportive relationships with women and with colleagues was important in their ability to cope well with the demands of their role'. These midwives learnt from women and 'the communication style associated with caseload midwifery was characterised by echoing and mirroring in conversational patterns and the posture of mothers and midwives'. Here again we see professionals with autonomy and ongoing relationships with clients behaving in ways which are enabling for those clients, facilitating open discussion and, in turn, receiving support from clients and colleagues. 'Developing the primacy of relationships took the place of developing professional distance' (Chapter 1).

Context is clearly important here. Midwives, in an ever-changing context over which they lack control, have little choice but to develop professional detachment and address their emotional labour to processing women through the system. In a smaller context, whether it be a group of caseholding colleagues (Chapter 1) or a birth centre (Kirkham 2003; Walsh 2006a, 2006b), trust can develop and midwives can invest their time so as to develop new skills in response to the needs of particular women.

Skilled facilitation can help midwives to develop emotional skills in relationship with clients and colleagues in hospitals (Kirkham 2004; Deery 2005) and in the smaller, potentially safer setting of birth centres (Jones 2000). Context and time are important in both cases. Kirsten Baker demonstrates in Chapter 12 how drama can provide the opportunity and the trigger for reflection, 'with intensity and in safety', on how 'existing emotional patterns can be changed' (Chapter 12). The forum theatre work is consciously political and faces the oppression that so many midwives experience at work in the central belief that 'where oppressive behaviour dominates, it will be reproduced' and that 'liberation from oppression must be done by and not on those experiencing it' (Chapter 12). In this way professional autonomy and enabling emotional relationships are fostered.

The building of our stories and the integration of experience is very important in learning positive emotional skills. Integration of their history of infertility into life stories during pregnancy is shown to have positive psychological outcomes for couples (Chapter 7). In Chapter 11, Ólöf Ásta Ólafsdóttir examines midwives' birth stories to reveal ways of knowing and working with emotions: 'connective knowing with women through the forming of relationships'. Listening and sharing are important in building emotional skills and intuition. Trust is important throughout this chapter, not least the midwife's trust in her own developing 'sense that comes'. In Chapter 12, Kirsten Baker describes midwives reforming their stories with the stimulus and opportunity provided by forum theatre. Respect for the stories of clients and professionals is evident throughout this book. Reproductive health is key in our life stories.

If we are to respect life stories, then the issue of how professionals use their own experience is central. Midwives describe their experience of breastfeeding (Chapter 6) and of pregnancy loss (Chapter 8) as helping their practice. The positive use of personal experience in relationships with clients requires considerable skill and insight into those experiences and this is rarely taught or formally developed. Susan Battersby has created a comprehensive model for professionals to review their personal experiences and perceptions of infant feeding (Battersby 2006 and Chapter 6). Such a review takes time and requires a safe setting with trusted colleagues. Personal reproductive experience is then integrated into professionals' stories to provide a resource rather than another occasion for detachment.

Coping with uncertainty is a major issue in reproductive health and is emotionally demanding. The medical response to uncertainty is one of control and intervention. Even when such an approach is advisable, uncertainty still has to be coped with emotionally. Some questions cannot be answered, or cannot be answered at the present time. In Chapters 8 and 9 we see ways of coping with longer-term uncertainty as to loss and future fertility. These ways of coping ranged from writing and creating mementos (Chapter 8) to distancing the problem by pushing it into the future (Chapter 9), since the knowledge needed to deal with it is not available at present. Detachment from the problem is clearly different from and probably more positive than detachment from people.

Coping with uncertainty in labour is the point where the tension between medical and midwifery models is most evident. In hospital the power of the medical model is paramount, and there is tremendous pressure to process women through the system. This requires emotional skills like those of air hostesses (Hochschild 1983) to process clients so as to ensure their state of mind is compliant with their medical management. Within such a situation 'therapeutic emotional labour' can improve clients' experience and bring professional job satisfaction (see Chapter 3). With increased pressures on staff time and standardisation of care, this becomes less possible and the potential for reciprocal engagement fades. Emotional labour then becomes 'hard graft' (Chapter 2), which is unrewarded; detachment is likely to follow: 'The only way to salvage a sense of self-esteem' then is 'to remove the self from the job'. Many do this by 'going into robot' (Hochschild 1983; 135). The air hostesses who did this 'describe it as a defence, they acknowledge that it is inadequate: their withdrawal irritates passengers', leading to further withdrawal. This is an unfortunate situation in flight, but a tragic one in birth.

The Way Forward

Key themes recur throughout this book, which indicate where change is needed. Structural change is required so that the potential for trusting relationships and emotional safety can be experienced by women and by their carers. This is wider than the issue of place of birth since hospitals are experienced as emotionally unsafe at other points in reproduction and known carers can achieve emotional safety within hospitals. Achievement of continuity of care for women and working in small teams for staff would allow relationships to develop and autonomy to be exercised. This can be achieved in many ways and is highly likely to result in good clinical outcomes, high client satisfaction and good staff retention. Such proposed change seems very logical and is underpinned by research but it runs counter to the major political trends which produced the care deficit: centralisation of services offering high tech but low care solutions. This therefore poses a major challenge which merits collective strategic debate by all those involved in women's reproductive health.

The care deficit and denial of dependence produce social and emotional impoverishment. Alliances are required to challenge this deficit in materially affluent nations. Social capital can be enhanced through the fostering of mutually supportive relationships. If such a supportive web of relationships is to be prioritised, it would be logical to have the newborn at its centre. As a political issue this would have to address time and resources for relationships around birth.

Personal change is needed as well as political change. Many of our defensive habits require much emotional labour but are counterproductive in the long term. Chapters in this book suggest ways in which we can learn more creative and sustainable forms of emotion work, and there other ways. Existing structures are not enabling midwives to focus their emotion work on building support networks and providing enabling care for women (see Chapters 8 and 10). Skilled facilitation and excellent role models are needed, as well as the opportunity to learn from them. 'Feeling cared for and about is probably the most potent and benign tonic there is' (Oakley 2001: vii). The nature of our emotional labour is an issue of quality of care for women and of occupational health for staff. We can all 'learn to do without' and work in ways which are mutually disempowering, or we can work more creatively. The choice is ours politically and educationally.

References

Battersby, S. (2006) Exploring attitudes towards infant feeding. In: V. Moran and F. Dykes (eds), *Maternal and Infant Nutrition and Nurture: Controversies and Challenges* (London: Quay Books).

Curtis, P., Ball, L. and Kirkham, M. (2006) Working together? Indices of division within the midwifery workforce, *British Journal of Midwifery*, 14(3): 138–41.

Deery, R. (2005) An action research study exploring midwives' support needs and the effect of group clinical supervision, *Midwifery*, 21: 161–76.

Deery, R. and Kirkham, M. (2007) Drained and dumped on: the generation and accumulation of emotional toxic waste in community midwifery. In: M. Kirkham (ed.), *Exploring the Dirty Side of Women's Health* (London: Routledge).

Dykes, F. (2006) *Breastfeeding in Hospital: Midwives, Mothers and the Production Line* (London: Routledge).

Edwards, N. (2005) *Birthing Autonomy: Women's Experiences of Planning Home Births* (Oxford: Routledge).

Glaser, B. and Strauss, A. L. (1968) *Time for Dying* (Chicago: Aldine).

Halldorsdóttir, S. and Karlsdóttir, S. I. (1996) Empowerment and discouragement: women's experience of caring and uncaring encounters during childbirth, *Health Care for Women International*, 17: 361–79.

Hochschild, A. R. (1983) *The Managed Heart: Commercialisation of Human Feeling* (Berkeley, CA: University of California Press).

Hochschild, A. R. (2003) *The Commercialisation of Intimate Life* (Berkeley, CA: University of California Press).

Hodnett, E. D. (2002) *Caregiver Support for Women During Childbirth (Cochrane Review)* (Oxford: The Cochrane Library Issue 4, update software).

Hunter, B. (2004) Conflicting ideologies as a source of emotion work in midwifery, *Midwifery*, 20: 261–72.

Hunter, B. (2005) Emotion work and boundary maintenance in hospital-based midwifery, *Midwifery*, 21: 253–66.

Hunter, B. (2006) The importance of reciprocity in relationships between community-based midwives and mothers, *Midwifery*, 22: 308–22.

Jones, O. (2000) Supervision in a midwife-managed birth centre. In: M. Kirkham (ed.), *Developments in the Supervision of Midwives* (Hale, Cheshire: Books for Midwives).

Kaplan, S. H., Greenfield, S., Gandek, B., Rogers, W. H. and Ware, J. E. (1996) Characteristics of physicians with participatory decision-making styles, *Annals of International Medicine*, 124(5): 497–504.

Kirkham, M. (1987) Basic supportive care in labour: interaction with and around women in labour. Unpublished PhD, University of Manchester, Faculty of Medicine.

Kirkham, M. (ed.) (2003) *Birth Centres: A Social Model for Maternity Care* (Oxford: Elsevier Science).

Kirkham, M. (2004) Midwives: praise and beyond, *The Practising Midwife*, 7(2): 20–1.

Kirkham, M. (2007) Traumatised midwives, *Aims Journal*, 19(1): 12–13.

Kirkham, M. and Morgan, R. K. (2006) *Why Midwives Return and their Subsequent Experience* (London: Department of Health; www.nhsemployers.org and www.rcm.org).

Kirkham, M. and Stapleton, H. (eds) (2001) *Informed Choice in Maternity Care: An Evaluation of Evidence-based Leaflets* (York: NHS Centre for Reviews and Dissemination).

Kirkham, M., Morgan, R. K. and Davies, C. (2006) *Why Midwives Stay* (London: Department of Health; www.nhsemployers.org and www.rcm.org).

Kirkham, M., Stapleton, H., Curtis, P. and Thomas, G. (2002a) Stereotyping as a professional defence mechanism, *British Journal of Midwifery*, 10(9): 509–13.

Kirkham, M., Stapleton, H., Thomas, G. and Curtis, P. (2002b) Checking not listening: how midwives cope, *British Journal of Midwifery*, 10(7): 447–50.

Leap, N. (2000) The less we do, the more we give. In: M. Kirkham (ed.), *The Midwife–Mother Relationship* (Basingstoke: Palgrave Macmillan).

Lundgren, I. and Dahlberg, K. (1998) Women's experience of pain during labour, *Midwifery*, 14(2): 105–10.

Mander, R. (2001) *Supportive Care and Midwifery* (Oxford: Blackwell).

Marx, K. (1st English edition 1887) *Capital* (Moscow: Progress Publishers).

Menzies, Lyth I. (1988) *Containing Anxiety in Institutions. Selected Essays*, vol. 1 (London: Free Association Books).

Murphy-Lawless, J. (1998) *Reading Birth and Death* (Cork: Cork University Press).

Oakley, A. (2001) Foreword to R. Mander, *Supportive Care and Midwifery* (Oxford: Blackwell).

Sandall, J. (1997) Midwives' burnout and continuity of care, *Midwifery*, 5(2): 106–11.

Sandall, J. (1998) Midwifery work, family life and wellbeing: a study of occupational change. Unpublished PhD, University of Surrey, Guildford.

Seigrist, J. (1996) Adverse health effects of high effort/low reward conditions, *Journal of Occupational Psychology*, 1(1): 27–41.

Seligman, M. E. P. (1975) *Helplessness: On Depression, Development and Death* (San Francisco, CA: Friedman).

Stapleton, H., Duerden, J. and Kirkham, M. (1998) *Evaluation of the Impact of the Supervision of Midwives on Professional Practice and the Quality of Midwifery Care* (London: English National Board).

Thompson, A. (1980) Planned or unplanned? Are midwives ready for the 1980s?, *Midwives Chronicle*, March: 68–72.

Walsh, D. J. (2006a) 'Nesting' and 'matrescence' as distinctive features of a free-standing birth centre in the UK, *Midwifery*, 22: 228–39.

Walsh, D. J. (2006b) Birth centres, community and social capital, *MIDIRS Midwifery Digest*, 16(1): 7–15.

Index